PHLEBOTOMY
PROCEDURES & PRACTICES

SECOND EDITION

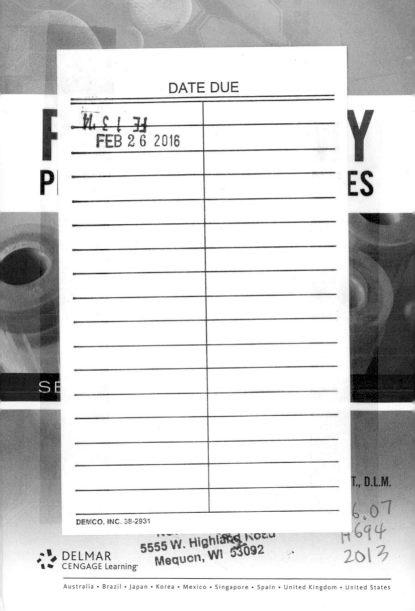

DATE DUE

F   Y
P   ES

SE

T., D.L.M.

6.07
H694
2013

5555 W. Highland Road
Mequon, WI 53092

DELMAR
CENGAGE Learning

Australia • Brazil • Japan • Korea • Mexico • Singapore • Spain • United Kingdom • United States

DELMAR
CENGAGE Learning·

Phlebotomy Procedures and Practices, 2nd Ed.
Lynn B. Hoeltke, M.B.A., M.T. (A.S.C.P.), P.B.T, D.L.M

Vice President, Editorial:
Dave Garza

Director of Learning Solutions: Matthew Kane

Associate Acquisitions Editor: Tom Stover

Managing Editor:
Marah Bellegarde

Senior Product Manager:
Laura J. Wood

Editorial Assistant: Anthony Souza

Vice President, Marketing:
Jennifer Ann Baker

Marketing Director:
Wendy E. Mapstone

Senior Marketing Manager:
Nancy Bradshaw

Marketing Coordinator:
Piper Huntington

Production Manager: Andrew Crouth

Content Project Manager:
Allyson Bozeth

Senior Art Director:
David Arsenault

Library of Congress Control Number: 2012931868

ISBN-13: 978-0-8400-2304-9

ISBN-10: 0-8400-2304-9

Delmar
5 Maxwell Drive
Clifton Park, NY 12065-2919
USA

Cengage Learning is a leading provider of customized learning solutions with office locations around the globe, including Singapore, the United Kingdom, Australia, Mexico, Brazil, and Japan. Locate your local office at: **international.cengage.com/region**

Cengage Learning products are represented in Canada by Nelson Education, Ltd.

To learn more about Delmar, visit **www.cengage.com/delmar**

Purchase any of our products at your local college store or at our preferred online store **www.cengagebrain.com**

Notice to the Reader

Printed in the United States of America
1 2 3 4 5 6 7 14 13 12

Contents

LIST OF PROCEDURES

Preface

This handbook on phlebotomy is written to teach phlebotomy skills to individuals who are already familiar with health care. Many individuals working in health care or taking health-care-related classes are discovering that they need to have a skill level in phlebotomy. Most phlebotomy textbooks contain information that the health care student or worker is already knowledgeable of. This book keeps it simple by explaining only phlebotomy and the procedures necessary to perform the task. This book is formatted for use in the practicum portion of phlebotomy classes, as the competency and training checklists are ideal for instructors and students to validate that each vital step is performed accurately and competently.

The book is very specific and concise in focusing on adult phlebotomy, microcollection, and infant heelsticks. It does not attempt to cover anatomy, information about laboratory tests, point of care testing, or performance of laboratory testing such as bleeding times. These are left to more complete textbooks, such as *The Complete Textbook of Phlebotomy, Fourth Edition*, by this author.

This book is to be used by health care workers needing specific information on phlebotomy procedures. Technical programs in medical assisting or nursing can use this as a supplemental text to teach basic phlebotomy. This book can be covered in several sessions rather than spending an entire semester on the subject. The instructor can use the complementary book, *The Complete Textbook of Phlebotomy, Fourth Edition*, and its instructor guide as a resource to answer student questions and develop test questions.

Hospitals and health care institutions that want to update their staff on the basics of phlebotomy can use this book as a reference to the newest and latest procedures and safety devices in use. Multiple pictures accompany procedures, making the learning experience easier. This handbook is an excellent reference guide to use for meeting competency training requirements.

Handbook Organization

This book is organized into three units. Rather than divide the book into chapters, the three units cover the three fundamentals of phlebotomy. Unit 1 focuses on customer service, the equipment used in phlebotomy, and how this equipment is used. Unit 2 directs the student in the venipuncture procedure and the variations that exist in obtaining blood. Unit 3 is dedicated to microcollection of blood.

New to the Second Edition

The entire book has been updated to be consistent with the newest Clinical Laboratory Standards Institute (CLSI) guidelines and standards. The CLSI is the main reference to how phlebotomy should be performed. Safety and proper biohazard precautions have been updated to the current standards.

The new edition of this book adds more information to answer questions that the health care associate will have about performing phlebotomy. More procedures have been added and updated to help the health care associate with step-by-step details to best perform his or her job. A new procedure, hand vein venipuncture by butterfly procedure, was added because many health care associates need this skill in difficult-to-draw patients.

Phlebotomy with infants has become the responsibility of the health care associate. Unit 3, Microcollection, was expanded with this need in mind. A section on obtaining a blood sample from babies was added and the procedure for infant heelsticks was added to cover this additional job requirement for many health care associates.

About the Author

Lynn B. Hoeltke, M.B.A., M.T. (A.S.C.P.), P.B.T., D.L.M., works as a supervisor for a leading hospital laboratory in the Midwest. He currently teaches phlebotomy as a career development program for entry-level positions in the laboratory. Lynn has more than 30 years' experience in various laboratory leadership roles. He has taught on the technical college level and has developed and taught a nursing-based program for a hospital. He has consulted with several nursing homes and laboratories in teaching phlebotomy techniques to their staff. He has published several magazine articles, has been a contributing author for *Comprehensive Medical Assisting*, and is author of *The Clinical Laboratory Manual Series: Phlebotomy* and *The Complete Textbook of Phlebotomy (4th Edition)*.

Reviewer Acknowledgments

Sherri Craddock, MLS (ASCP)
Assistant Professor
Pierpont Community and Technical College
Fairmont, WV

Dr. C. Thomas Somma
Associate Professor
School of Medical Laboratory and Radiation Sciences
Old Dominion University

Learning Objectives

Unit 1

After studying this unit, the participant will be able to:

1. Describe the manner in which the patient affects the success of the venipuncture.
2. Describe the three different formed elements in the blood.
3. Differentiate between serum and plasma.
4. State the manner in which anticoagulants prevent coagulation.
5. Name the anticoagulant, if any, associated with color-coded tubes.
    a. Gray
    b. Light blue
    c. Lavender
    d. Green
    e. Gold
    f. Red/black
    g. White
6. State the anticoagulant that requires a 1:9 anticoagulant-to-blood ratio and why this is essential.
7. Name the types of tubes that produce a serum sample.
8. State the purpose of the following additives/tubes:
    a. Serum separation tubes (gel tubes)
    b. Trace element

Unit 2

After studying this unit, the participant will be able to:

1. Explain the implications of not labeling samples correctly.
2. List all information that must be on the label of a sample submitted for laboratory testing.
3. State a way to prevent hemoconcentration.
4. List methods to prevent hemolysis during blood collection.
5. Discuss three blood collection alternatives when a patient has an intravenous line running.
6. Describe how much of a discard is pulled from a vascular access device.
7. Explain the single most important way to prevent the spread of infection in a hospital.
8. List four common venipuncture sites.
9. List four techniques that can be used to make a vein easier to feel.
10. State the maximum number of times a venipuncture should be attempted by one person.
11. Explain the importance of proper skin antisepsis in blood culture collection.
12. Explain proper blood culture bottle preparation.
13. Define the following terms:
    a. Cellular elements
    b. Buffy coat
    c. Hemoconcentration
    d. Glycolysis
14. Describe how to successfully perform venipuncture by demonstrating correct:
    a. Selection of equipment
    b. Selection of the appropriate site
    c. Preparation of the site
    d. Venipuncture of the patient

    e. Collection of multiple tubes

    f. Care of the site after collection

15. Indicate the correct order of drawing evacuated tubes and blood culture bottles for venous blood collection.

16. Indicate the three basic methods of collecting a peripheral blood sample.

Unit 3

After studying this unit, the participant will be able to:

1. Describe capillary puncture equipment and proper depth of cut for this equipment.

2. Describe the composition of capillary puncture blood.

3. Describe what warming of the capillary puncture site accomplishes.

4. Determine the safest area of a finger to puncture.

5. Explain the key to an acceptable capillary puncture sample.

6. Explain why hemolysis is more likely in capillary puncture blood.

7. State why the first drop of blood is wiped away during capillary puncture.

8. Explain the order of draw for microcollection.

9. Describe the proper procedure for collection of blood from an infant.

UNIT 1
VENIPUNCTURE PRINCIPLES

Focusing on the Patient

*T*he emphasis in health care is on seeking ways to reduce costs, shorten patient days, and maintain quality care, all while treating the patient as a customer. This customer must be so satisfied with the care that he or she will come back and recommend the health care facility to his or her friends. This is nothing new to health care, but pressures from third-party payers and government regulation have challenged all health care facilities in their ability to cut costs and still satisfy patients. One way to blend these two demands of reducing costs and enhancing patient recognition of care is to use patient-focused care. The most effective method of achieving patient-focused care and reducing costs is to treat the patient as quickly as possible and return that patient to the security and safety of his or her home. The faster the patient can be sent out of the hospital or health care facility, the faster that bed can be refilled with a new patient. The same holds true for outpatients. The faster patients can be serviced, the sooner they can receive appropriate care or diagnosis and the sooner they can return to a normal life. This is the basic economics of any retail store. The more items a store sells in a specific amount of time, the more revenue is generated. The more patients that come in and out of the health care facility, the stronger the organization is financially.

This type of economics does not negate the needs of the patient. The stronger an organization is financially, the better equipment, specialists, and care the organization can offer the patient. Most patients would rather walk into a modern, clean, and well-maintained building than a building that is in disrepair. The caregiver must keep in mind that each patient is an individual with specific needs. No matter how large the health care organization, when the caregiver is with a patient, that patient should feel that he or she is the only patient that organization is working with that day.

The laboratory plays an integral part in how long it takes the patient to receive proper care. If it takes hours or days to complete necessary testing, the physician is waiting on results and the patient is waiting on treatment. A key delay in result reporting is in the beginning of the testing cycle. This delay is caused by the preexamination (preanalytical) time it takes to obtain the sample. To speed the process of patient testing, the samples need to be drawn at the critical moments in that patient's time in the hospital. It takes time to get a phlebotomist up to the nursing unit. The exact moment when that patient should have been tested may have passed. It would be nice to have one phlebotomist for every 10 to 15 patients. That way whenever a sample needs to be drawn, a phlebotomist would be right there to provide instant phlebotomy. Unfortunately, it would not be cost effective to hire that many phlebotomists. This ratio of patients to phlebotomist can be obtained if the definition of phlebotomist is expanded. As hospitals explore new ways to develop this patient-focused care, the laboratory is often asked to no longer do phlebotomy but to relinquish this duty to the nursing staff. This practice of using associates from the nursing floors and not the laboratory is called decentralized phlebotomy.

A mix of reactions from both laboratorians and nurses is seen when this type of shift in duties occurs. The phlebotomy staff is worried about losing their jobs. In addition, there is concern about the quality of the samples that will be received. The nurses often voice concern because they are being asked to do one more job they do not have time for. These are very valid concerns that need to be addressed before any hospital embarks on the task of using nurses as phlebotomists.

Patient-focused care directs our attention to the patient and what would be best for the patient's comfort. While doing this, the physician and health care facility must get the patient well as rapidly as possible and send the patient home as a satisfied individual.

This book focuses on the methods that phlebotomists can use to make patients' experiences as comfortable and efficient as possible. Patients are generally fearful of having their blood drawn. Surveys of patients often reveal that the procedure patients disliked the most was having their blood drawn. This fear is universal, without reference to who drew the blood.

Communicating with the patient and putting the patient at ease are essential to successful venipuncture. Positive feedback from patients about their experience always stresses how they "did not feel a thing" when their blood was drawn and how the person drawing their blood was "friendly" and "professional." Focusing on the patient during the encounter and communicating with the patient in a friendly, caring manner are keys to compassionate care.

Customer Service

Customer service is composed of many facets that can either make a patient appreciative of quality service or angry because the patient's entire needs were not met. The phlebotomist who meets the patient's needs is the phlebotomist providing the best customer service. Consistently meeting and exceeding these expectations is difficult.

The phlebotomist works with both external and internal customers. An external customer for the phlebotomist is the patient. But for the phlebotomist, the patient is not the only customer. There are many internal customers, such as the nurse caring for the patient, the physician, the family of the patient, and so on. Each customer has an interest in what the phlebotomist does. The patient wants a caring, nearly pain-free procedure. The physician wants timely, quality results. The family of the patient wants a caring, quality person taking care of the family member. The family also wants someone who keeps them informed and does not treat them as if they are in the way. A simple question to ask is "How would you like to be treated if you were the patient?"

To achieve quality service, the phlebotomist must meet three expectations:

1. Know what the customer wants.
2. Determine whether or not the customer is getting the service he or she wants.
3. Continuously take action to satisfy the customer.

Patient Satisfaction

Keeping the patient satisfied is the primary role of the phlebotomist. The customer expects and demands a quality encounter in the phlebotomy experience. The customer will tell other customers that the phlebotomist was excellent at drawing blood, was very friendly, and that the wait was not too long. The patient does not care about the details or the problems of the day; the patient only cares about being treated with compassion and having a quality sample obtained. Each patient should be treated like a guest in your home. Treat each patient as if he or she is the most important patient of the day, and give that patient individualized attention.

The patient can come into the facility dissatisfied. This is a challenge for the phlebotomist to "read" the customer and improve the customer's satisfaction. Factors affecting the customer's satisfaction could include a previous negative experience, personality characteristics, high expectations, or the time the patient allowed for the laboratory visit. If the reality did not match what the patient expected, the patient's experience will be negative. For example, a negative expectation for the patient is created if the minimum time it takes for a patient to register and get blood drawn is 15 minutes but the patient expected the process to be completed in 5 minutes. For this patient to become satisfied, the patient needs to allow more time to get his or her blood drawn. Helping the patient understand the process means taking the time to communicate. The more information the patient is given, the better the patient will understand how long the process takes. A patient usually is not concerned about the time if he or she is getting attention during that time.

Universal Precautions, Body Substance Isolation, and Standard Precautions

Universal precautions were developed in 1985 by the Centers for Disease Control and Prevention (CDC) as a response to the increase of acquired immunodeficiency syndrome (AIDS) and hepatitis B, both blood-borne diseases. Any patient has the potential to be infected with these **blood-borne pathogens.** Universal precautions assume that all blood and most body fluids are potentially infectious. Because it is impossible to know if a patient is infectious, the health care worker must treat all patients with universal precautions for infection.

Techniques for handling a patient's body fluids evolved into a system called **body substance isolation (BSI).** Like universal precautions, BSI assumed that each patient had the potential to spread disease through body substances. The key change was the requirement that gloves be worn when in contact with any body substance.

In 1996 the CDC revised universal precautions and released a new set of guidelines, still in use today, called **standard precautions.** These precautions create a first tier of precautions for all patients regardless of their diagnosis or infectious status.

Standard precautions combine many of the basic principles of universal precautions with techniques from BSI. Standard precautions maintain that personal protective equipment and barrier controls must be worn for contact with all body fluids whether or not blood is visible. The goal of standard precautions is to reduce the risk of transmission of microorganisms from both recognized and unrecognized sources of infection. Five main points must be followed in standard precautions.

Handwashing and Disinfecting

Handwashing is a work practice control that is incorporated into the phlebotomist's work habits to prevent the spread of infection. Handwashing is the single most important way to prevent the spread of

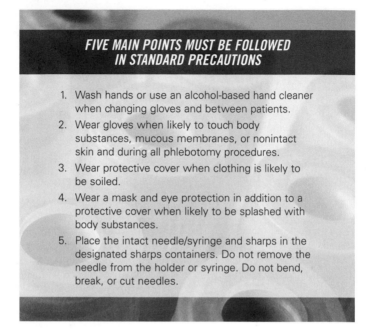

FIVE MAIN POINTS MUST BE FOLLOWED IN STANDARD PRECAUTIONS

1. Wash hands or use an alcohol-based hand cleaner when changing gloves and between patients.
2. Wear gloves when likely to touch body substances, mucous membranes, or nonintact skin and during all phlebotomy procedures.
3. Wear protective cover when clothing is likely to be soiled.
4. Wear a mask and eye protection in addition to a protective cover when likely to be splashed with body substances.
5. Place the intact needle/syringe and sharps in the designated sharps containers. Do not remove the needle from the holder or syringe. Do not bend, break, or cut needles.

infection. Hands must be washed after each patient contact or blood and body fluid exposure, even when gloves are used. Hands must be washed under running water with soap and vigorous rubbing. When rinsing the soap off, the water should flow from the wrists to the fingertips. Handwashing is the method of choice for removing any surface bacteria from the skin. See Procedure 1.1. Hands must be washed after removing gloves because the gloves may have defects, allowing contaminants (bacteria or viruses) to penetrate the imperfections of the gloves.

Procedure 1.1 illustrates the proper method for medical asepsis handwashing.

Alcohol-based hand cleaners are often used to clean the skin surface in place of handwashing. Alcohol-based hand cleaners are chemical

PROCEDURE 1.1 Medical Asepsis Handwashing

Principle:

To clean the hands with the use of soap and running water and reduce the number of organisms on the hands and wrists. The purpose is to decrease the transfer of organisms from a source to a susceptible host.

Materials:

- Sink with running water, preferably with foot-operated controls or hand-sensor automatic dispenser
- Soap from a foot-operated container or a pump container (bar soap is discouraged)
- Disposable paper towels
- Nailstick and/or brush

Procedure:

1. Remove all rings, watches, and other jewelry to prevent them from harboring microorganisms.
2. Have disposable towels ready or use an automatic towel dispenser.
3. Stand back from the sink so that you or your clothing does not touch the sink.
4. Turn on the water with the foot pedal or with a disposable towel if not foot controlled. Temperature should be lukewarm (Figure 1.1).
5. Wet hands under the running water. Be careful to not touch the sides of the sink (Figure 1.2).

continues

PROCEDURE 1.1 Medical Asepsis Handwashing
continued

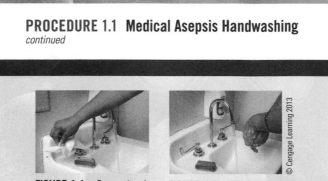

© Cengage Learning 2013

FIGURE 1.1 *Prepare towels for use; turn on the water.*

FIGURE 1.2 *Wet hands under the running water.*

6. Apply soap and lather well. The lather and friction scrubbing action will remove dirt and dead skin. Scrub between fingers and around fingernails (Figure 1.3). Use a nailstick and a brush during the first handwashing of each day or when your hands become excessively soiled. Continue to scrub for at least 15 to 20 seconds. Some facilities will have a specific minimum time to scrub (Figures 1.4 and 1.5).

7. Rinse hands with the water flowing downward off the fingertips. This will rinse the contaminated water off the fingertips and not onto the forearms (Figure 1.6).

8. Complete the washing process again if this is the first handwashing of the day. (Repeat steps 6 and 7.)

9. Dry hands and wrists with the disposable towels.

10. Turn off the water with the disposable towels if the sink is not foot controlled or electronically controlled.

continues

PROCEDURE 1.1 Medical Asepsis Handwashing
continued

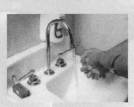

FIGURE 1.3   *Apply soap and lather well.*

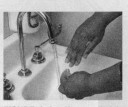

FIGURE 1.4   *Use a nailstick under the fingernails.*

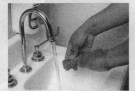

FIGURE 1.5   *Use a brush to clean around fingernails.*

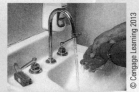

FIGURE 1.6   *Rinse hands with water flowing downward off hands and fingertips.*

© Cengage Learning 2013

solutions that reduce the number of bacteria on the skin surface. Handwashing and the use of hand cleaners both reduce bacteria and viruses but do not totally eliminate them.

Alcohol-based hand cleaners often are acceptable in place of handwashing. The hand cleaners have become widely accepted because even when running water is available, people are more likely to use hand cleaner than to wash hands. It is very simple, when going from one patient to another, to rub hand cleaner into your hands. This takes less time than a proper handwashing. Because most people do not spend sufficient time washing their hands, the hand cleaner does a more thorough job. Handwashing must be done if there is visible blood on the hands or if you are prepping for a sterile procedure.

Disinfecting of hard surfaces such as countertops is accomplished to produce a nearly sterile surface. Disinfecting solutions are too harsh for the skin, but they can kill up to 100 percent of the contaminants. Total sterilization of human skin is not acceptable because of chemical harshness. Multiple solutions are commercially available for the sterilization of work surfaces. Commercially available solutions usually come in spray bottles or towelette wipes. The least expensive and most effective is 10 percent household bleach. This can be made by adding 1 part bleach to 10 parts water and then either spraying it or wiping it on the surface. Bleach solution must be made daily. Whenever a 10 percent bleach solution is made, the container must be marked with the time and date the solution was made. If it has been more than 24 hours, the solution must be discarded and a new solution made with a new date and time documented on the container.

Gloves

There are three reasons for wearing gloves in patient care:

1. Sterile gloves prevent health care workers from transmitting their own microflora to the patient, such as during surgery or wound cleansing.
2. Gloves prevent the transmission of microorganisms from one patient to another.
3. Gloves prevent the phlebotomist from becoming infected with what is infecting the patient.

Always remove gloves according to Procedure 1.2.

PROCEDURE 1.2 Removing Contaminated Gloves

Principle:
To remove gloves after use to avoid contamination of the phlebotomist. The purpose is to decrease the transfer of organisms from a patient to a phlebotomist or phlebotomist to a patient.

Materials:
- Gloves sized to properly fit
- Biohazard waste container

Procedure:
1. Hold hands out in front of the body.
2. Grasp the palm of one hand, and pull down on the glove to pull the glove inside out. A right-handed person would naturally pull the palm of the left hand. Do not touch the bare skin or the contaminated glove (Figures 1.7, 1.8, and 1.9).
3. The hand still having the glove on should then hold the removed glove (Figure 1.10).
4. Contain the inverted glove completely in the gloved hand (Figure 1.11).
5. Insert two fingers of the ungloved hand under the cuff of the glove of the other hand (Figure 1.12).
6. Pull down on this glove to turn the glove inside out (Figure 1.13).
7. This will invert the glove and contain the other glove inside the inverted glove (Figure 1.14).

continues

PROCEDURE 1.2 Removing Contaminated Gloves
continued

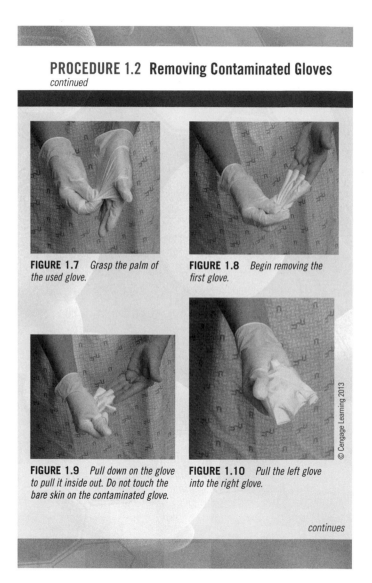

FIGURE 1.7   *Grasp the palm of the used glove.*

FIGURE 1.8   *Begin removing the first glove.*

FIGURE 1.9   *Pull down on the glove to pull it inside out. Do not touch the bare skin on the contaminated glove.*

FIGURE 1.10   *Pull the left glove into the right glove.*

© Cengage Learning 2013

continues

PROCEDURE 1.2 Removing Contaminated Gloves
continued

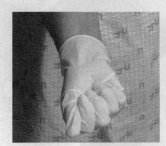

FIGURE 1.11   *Hold the glove in the right hand.*

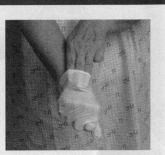

FIGURE 1.12   *Insert two fingers under the cuff of the other glove.*

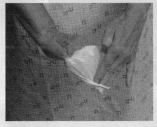

FIGURE 1.13   *Use the two ungloved fingers to pull the glove inside out.*

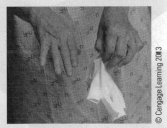

FIGURE 1.14   *One glove is now inside the other.*

© Cengage Learning 2013

8. Dispose of the gloves in a biohazard waste container.
9. Wash hands with running water.

BLOOD COMPONENTS

The blood of an adult consists of about 45 percent formed elements. The formed cellular elements are **erythrocytes** (red blood cells), **leukocytes** (white blood cells), and **thrombocytes** (platelets) (Figure 1.15).

Generally, 2 milliliters of blood yields about 1 milliliter of fluid. In the body, the liquid portion is called plasma. When the blood is removed from the body and allowed to clot, the liquid portion is called serum.

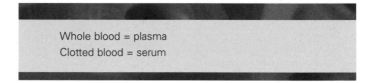

Whole blood = plasma
Clotted blood = serum

The clot contains all the formed elements intertwined together in a fibrin mass. Blood flowing through the body contains a substance called fibrinogen. Once the blood leaves the body, the fibrinogen turns into fibrin. This fibrin is like a sticky spider web and traps the formed elements into the fibrin mass called a clot. The clot then contracts, and the liquid (serum) portion is extracted. This serum is

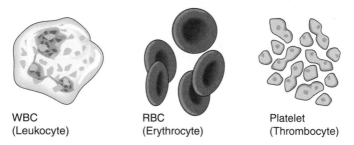

WBC   RBC   Platelet
(Leukocyte)   (Erythrocyte)   (Thrombocyte)

FIGURE 1.15   *Formed cellular elements of the peripheral blood.*
© Cengage Learning 2013

a clear, straw-colored liquid that is used for many of the tests done in the laboratory.

Different tests require different types of blood samples. Some tests require a serum sample. The tube used will be one that allows the blood to clot, such as a red-, gold-, or red/black-stoppered tube. Other tests require a whole-blood or plasma sample and need to be drawn in a sample container that does not allow it to clot. To prevent clotting of the blood, the tube contains an anticoagulant. An anticoagulant is a chemical substance that prevents coagulation by removing calcium and forming calcium salts or by inhibiting the conversion of prothrombin to thrombin. Both calcium and thrombin are part of the coagulation cascade (Figure 1.16). The coagulation cascade is like a staircase in which a ball is bounced down each step. The blood clots when the ball reaches the bottom of the stairs. If a step is taken away, the ball does not reach the bottom of the stairs and the blood does not clot. This staircase contains many steps. These steps consist of

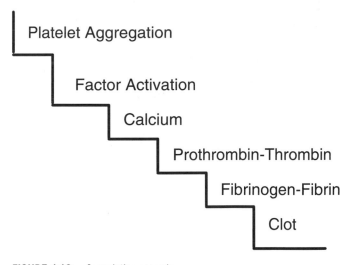

Platelet Aggregation

Factor Activation

Calcium

Prothrombin-Thrombin

Fibrinogen-Fibrin

Clot

FIGURE 1.16   *Coagulation cascade.*
© Cengage Learning 2013

different chemicals and factors that are required for a person's blood to clot. A person with a bleeding disorder has one of the factors missing or is physically unable to use a needed chemical. One disorder of this type is hemophilia. The patient can temporarily overcome this bleeding disorder by receiving an appropriate factor. A person with hemophilia has one of the steps in the staircase missing. By giving the person with hemophilia a factor such as factor VIII, the step is rebuilt and clotting occurs.

This process of clotting can be stopped in the test tube. A tube containing an anticoagulant removes one of the steps to the staircase, meaning the blood will not clot. The anticoagulant prevents clotting depending on the anticoagulant used. The anticoagulants used are oxalates, citrates, ethylenediaminetetraacetic acid (EDTA), and heparin.

In the process of going down the stairs, six basic steps occur.

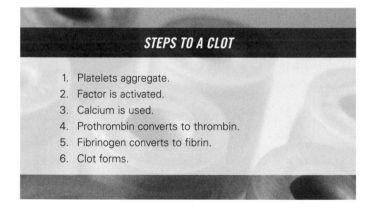

STEPS TO A CLOT

1. Platelets aggregate.
2. Factor is activated.
3. Calcium is used.
4. Prothrombin converts to thrombin.
5. Fibrinogen converts to fibrin.
6. Clot forms.

When the blood samples are centrifuged, a layering of the elements of the blood occurs (Figure 1.17). To produce a plasma sample, the blood has to be prevented from clotting. In an anticoagulated tube of blood that has been centrifuged, the formed elements and plasma are layered according to weight. The bottom layer contains erythrocytes; then there is a thin layer called the buffy coat, which contains a mixture of leukocytes and thrombocytes. On top of these layers

Anticoagulated Blood   Non-anticoagulated Blood

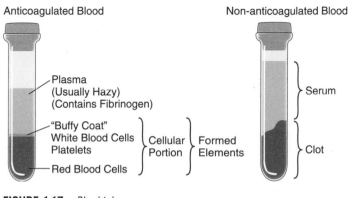

FIGURE 1.17   *Blood tubes.*
© Cengage Learning 2013

is the plasma layer. The plasma contains fibrinogen and usually is slightly hazy. To produce a serum sample, the blood must be allowed to clot. This usually takes at least 15 to 30 minutes. The serum forms on the top layer with the clot on the bottom. The main difference between serum and plasma is that plasma contains fibrinogen and serum does not.

Anticoagulants

Anticoagulants work on two principles. The anticoagulant either precipitates/removes the calcium or stops the prothrombin-to-thrombin reaction from progressing. Various tubes are available with different anticoagulants for various laboratory testing. The most common tube types are listed in Figure 1.18.

Gray-stoppered Tubes

Gray-stoppered tubes contain potassium oxalate in combination with another weak glycolytic agent, sodium fluoride. The anticoagulant combination of potassium oxalate and sodium fluoride works by

Tube Stopper Color	Additive	Additive Action	Laboratory Use	Laboratory Department
Gray	Potassium oxalate/sodium fluoride or sodium fluoride/EDTA	Binds calcium/ stabilizes glucose values	Glucose testing	Chemistry
Light Blue	Sodium citrate	Binds calcium	Used for coagulation studies; tubes must be filled to the proper level	Coagulation
Lavender	Ethylene diaminetetra - acetic acid (EDTA)	Binds calcium	Hematology testing	Hematology
Green	Lithium heparin or sodium heparin	Inhibits prothrombin- to-thrombin formation	Plasma determinations in chemistry	STAT Chemistry
Yellow	Solution A or B (ACD)	Binds calcium	DNA, paternity testing, HLA phenotyping, and immunohematology studies	Chemistry or Blood Bank
Yellow	Sodium polyanthol sulfonate (SPS)	Binds calcium	Used to collect blood cultures	Microbiology
Pink	EDTA	Binds calcium	Immunohematology testing	Blood Bank
Orange	Thrombin clot activator	Clot forms	Stat serum testing	STAT Chemistry
White (pearl top)	EDTA	Binds calcium	Polymerase chain reaction (PCR) or DNA amplification techniques	Molecular Diagnostics

FIGURE 1.18 *Tube guide.*   (*continues*)
© Cengage Learning 2013

Royal Blue	Sodium heparin, EDTA, or no additive	Inhibits thrombin formation, binds calcium or clots	Plasma or serum toxicology	Special Chemistry
Red	Glass tube— no additive Plastic tube— clot activators	Clot forms	Serum for various tests	Blood Bank, Immunology, Drug Testing
SST, Gold or Red/ Black	Clot activators, gel separator	Clot forms	Serum for various tests	Chemistry

FIGURE 1.18   *Tube guide. (continued)*
© Cengage Learning 2013

precipitating out the calcium in the blood and therefore stopping the coagulation cascade. The sodium fluoride's primary function is not as an anticoagulant but as a glycolytic inhibitor. The fluoride preserves the glucose in the blood sample by inhibiting the enzymes involved in breakdown of the glucose (glycolysis). As a blood sample sits without the fluoride, the glucose is broken down at a rate of around 7 percent per hour. A sample that was drawn from a patient and left to sit will have a falsely lower glucose value. This can be pictured as little men opening their mouths and devouring the glucose molecules. Over time there would be no glucose molecules left. The fluoride keeps these men from opening their mouths and helps preserve the glucose.

Often there is a delay between the time a sample is drawn from a patient and when it makes it to the laboratory to be tested. The physician wants to monitor the glucose of the patient at the time the sample is drawn. If the glucose is allowed to decrease in the sample, the results at the time of testing would indicate that the patient had a glucose value less than actual. The patient would then be falsely treated for a low glucose. The way to prevent this is to draw samples to be tested for glucose in a gray-stoppered tube if there is to be a delay in testing. This tube is used for glucose tests such as fasting blood sugar (FBS), random blood glucose, postprandial glucose, and glucose tolerance tests.

Light Blue–stoppered Tubes

Light blue–stoppered tubes contain the anticoagulant sodium citrate. Sodium citrate prevents the coagulation by binding calcium in a non-ionized form. The sodium citrate anticoagulant most widely used is 3.2 percent buffered sodium citrate (0.105M). Citrate is used primarily in coagulation studies. It is critical that the light blue–stoppered tubes be filled to their proper level for accurate patient results. A ratio of one part anticoagulant to nine parts blood must be maintained. If a tube is only half filled, the ratio will be off and the results will be invalid. The anticoagulant in the tube prevents the blood from clotting by binding the calcium. To test the blood for coagulation studies, the blood is centrifuged to produce a plasma sample. An aliquot of this plasma sample combines with other chemicals to restart the coagulation process and produce a clot. The time it takes for a visible clot to form is the result for the coagulation study. There are normal time ranges for this clotting to occur, and an abnormal result falls outside these ranges. Tests using the light blue–stoppered tube to detect clotting problems include prothrombin time (PT), activated partial thromboplastin time (aPTT), D-dimer, fibrin split products, factor assays, and fibrinogen assay.

Lavender-stoppered Tubes

Lavender-stoppered tubes contain the anticoagulant EDTA. This anticoagulant also binds the calcium to prevent coagulation. EDTA comes in two forms, either liquid (K3EDTA) or powder (K2EDTA). Liquid EDTA is found in the glass tubes, and powdered EDTA is found in the plastic tubes. Dipotassium EDTA is now the anticoagulant recommended by the International Council for Standardization in Hematology (ICSH) and the Clinical and Laboratory Standards Institute for hematology procedures. Dipotassium EDTA is recommended because it preserves cell morphology for complete blood cell counts (CBCs) and differential blood smears and provides stable microhematocrit results. Other anticoagulants distort the size and shape of the cells. This distortion often makes it appear that a disease process is occurring in the patient, when it is actually the effects of the anticoagulant. Tests using the lavender-stoppered tube are CBC, hemoglobin (Hgb), hematocrit (Hct), and hemoglobin A_1C.

Green-stoppered Tubes

Up to this point, all the anticoagulants discussed are those that prevent coagulation by precipitating or binding the calcium in the blood. Green-stoppered tubes contain heparin, which stops coagulation by inhibiting the conversion of prothrombin to thrombin and thus inhibiting the following stages that lead to a clot. What has occurred is that no fibrin is formed to cause a clot. Heparin is a naturally occurring substance that is present in most of our tissues but at low levels. Because of this it has the least effect on clinical chemistry tests of all the anticoagulants. It produces the least stress on erythrocytes and minimizes hemolysis.

Heparin is the anticoagulant of choice for pH determinations, electrolyte studies, and arterial blood gases. Heparin comes in three forms: lithium heparin, sodium heparin, and ammonium heparin. The lithium heparin and sodium heparin are the heparins found in evacuated tubes. Before drawing a test with a heparin tube, you must know what type of heparin is acceptable. Heparin is not acceptable for blood samples that may be stored for more than 48 hours before testing. After this time, heparinized blood will slowly begin to clot, forming small fibrin strands.

Solutions A and B (ACD)

Yellow-stoppered tubes, labeled as Solution A or Solution B, contain variations of a mixture of trisodium citrate, citric acid, and dextrose. They are used for DNA and paternity testing, human leukocyte antigen (HLA) phenotyping, and some immunohematology studies.

Sodium Polyanethol Sulfonate (SPS)

A yellow-stoppered tube that does not contain citrate is used for collecting blood culture samples. This tube looks the same as the two previous tubes except it contains the additive sodium polyanethol sulfonate (SPS). The main function of the SPS tube is to allow bacteria to grow so they can be cultured. SPS (1) inhibits the phagocytosis of the bacteria by the white blood cells (WBCs); (2) inhibits serum complement, which would destroy the bacteria; and (3) inhibits certain antibiotics in the case of a patient already on an antibiotic. The yellow-stoppered tube can be confusing in that there are multiple types of yellow-stoppered tubes with specific uses. The phlebotomist must read the label before using one of these tubes to ensure that the proper tube with the proper additive is used.

Pink-stoppered Tubes

Pink-stoppered tubes contain the anticoagulant EDTA, which binds the calcium to prevent coagulation and is the same anticoagulant as the K2EDTA in the lavender-stoppered tubes. This tube is made for immunohematology testing and is designed with a special crossmatch label for required information by the American Association of Blood Banks (AABB).

Orange-stoppered Tubes

Thrombin is a clot activator used for STAT (emergency) testing. The thrombin is within the tube to hasten the clotting process faster than silica particles. These tubes usually have an orange stopper. Most chemistry tests that can be performed on serum can use this tube as a substitute.

White-stoppered Tubes

White-stoppered tubes (also know as pearl top) contain EDTA as an anticoagulant and also a gel to separate the plasma from the cells. A sample for EDTA plasma can be collected in this tube, the tube centrifuged, and then frozen without pouring off the plasma into a separate tube. This is especially helpful in working with patients who are positive for human immunodeficiency virus (HIV). Processing the blood without a need to open the tube provides greater safety for the phlebotomist. This tube is used for molecular diagnostic tests such as polymerase chain reaction (PCR) or branched DNA amplification techniques.

Royal Blue–stoppered Tubes

Drawing blood for trace elements is when blood is being tested for heavy metals such as arsenic or lead. The only difference in the collection is that the blood must be collected in a special metal-free tube. These are usually royal blue–stoppered tubes that may or may not contain an anticoagulant. The tube and rubber stoppers have been specially refined to be metal free. Traces of metal in the routinely used evacuated tube may leach into the sample and give the patient a falsely elevated heavy metal value. The tubes have sodium heparin, EDTA, or no additive and a green, lavender, or red band on the label to indicate the type of additive or no additive in the tube. Therefore, the phlebotomist must read the label carefully to verify the type of tube being used.

Glass Red-stoppered Tubes

The glass red-stoppered tube is the traditional tube used when a serum sample from a clotted tube of blood is needed. The glass red-stoppered tube has no anticoagulants. Most blood collection tubes have a silicon coating on the interior surface of the tube. This silicon fills the microscopically rough surface of the glass. Glass may feel smooth to the touch, but it has a rough surface that cells can stick to. The silicon fills these cracks and crevasses and prevents the cells from adhering to the glass surface. This reduces the chance for hemolysis and makes the sides slicker so the cells can centrifuge to the bottom of the tube faster. These tubes have a red stopper, red/black stopper, or gold stopper (Hemogard brand tube), depending on the manufacturer.

Plastic Red-stoppered Tubes

The glass surface of a tube used for serum testing activates clot formation in the tube. Some glass serum tubes have a clot activator added to speed the clotting process. A plastic tube will not activate a clot; therefore, a clot activator must be added to each tube during manufacture of the tube. The clot activator added to the tubes is a silica coating on the sides of the tubes. Various additives are added to the tubes to improve the quality of the sample. These additives are

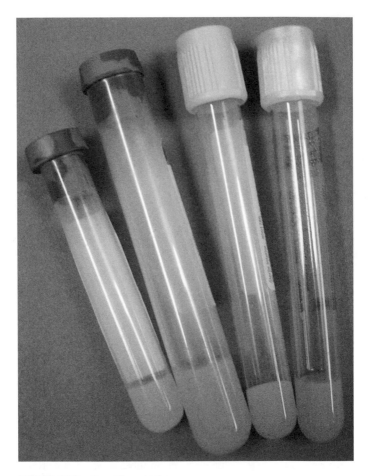

FIGURE 1.19 *Separator gel tubes.*
© Cengage Learning 2013

not anticoagulants or preservatives but are used to improve sample quality or accelerate sample processing.

Gel Separator

Serum and plasma tubes can also be purchased with a thixotropic separator gel (Figure 1.19). This gel is an inert material that undergoes a temporary change in viscosity during centrifugation. It has a density that is intermediate to cells/clot and plasma/serum. When centrifuged, the gel moves up the sides of the tube and engulfs the cells/clot; an interface of gel forms that separates the cells/clot from the plasma/serum (Figure 1.20). These tubes are often called SSTs, for serum separator tubes, or PSTs, for plasma separator tubes.

The separator gel helps preserve the constituents of the serum/plasma so that the chemistries being tested for will not deteriorate if testing cannot be done immediately. The gel preserves the serum/plasma without the need to aliquot the serum/plasma into a separate plain tube. This provides a savings in extra tubes and makes processing the tube faster and safer. The gel allows the tube to be transported without the cells mixing with the serum/plasma. The gel traps the cells in the bottom of the tube. The use of separator gel tubes is limited in that they cannot be used for some drug testing, blood bank, or testing for cold agglutinins or cryoglobulins.

More information can be found on the tubes by searching Web sites such as www.bd.com/vacutainer or www.vacuette.com.

Why So Many Choices in Types of Tubes

Many choices need to be made to collect the correct sample when drawing blood from a patient. There are many different tubes to select from, and different tests require different tubes. Trying to understand why one tube cannot do all the testing often gets confusing. This was explained to some degree in the section on anticoagulants.

Only two types of tubes are collected from a patient: tubes that clot, and tubes that have an anticoagulant in the tube to prevent clotting.

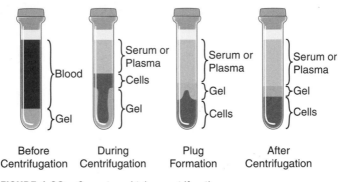

FIGURE 1.20 *Separator gel tubes: centrifugation process.*
© Cengage Learning 2013

The clotted tube produces liquid serum, and the anticoagulant tube produces liquid plasma. For a tube to clot, the blood in the tube must go through the six steps mentioned earlier:

1. Platelet clumping (platelet aggregation)
2. Factor activation
3. Calcium present to activate clotting
4. Prothrombin converting to thrombin
5. Fibrinogen converting to fibrin
6. Final clot formation

Blood placed in a red-stoppered tube goes through all these steps. Tubes with gel serum separator (SSTs) go through the same steps. The gel in the tube works to separate the serum from the clot. The gel tube can be used for most serum tests but has been known to absorb some of the drugs being tested, so it is not used for drug monitoring. Even though both types of tubes produce a serum sample, they each have their own reason for being collected.

Anticoagulant tubes are collected when nonclotted whole blood or plasma is needed. Each tube is unique in its use in testing, and the anticoagulants work differently. Any blood placed in these tubes will try

Tube Type	Anticoagulant	Prevents clotting by:
Lavender stoppered	EDTA	Removing the calcium to stop the coagulation process
Gray stoppered	Potassium oxalate/ sodium fluoride	Potassium oxalate: removing the calcium Sodium fluoride: preserving the glucose
Light-blue stoppered	Sodium citrate	Binding the calcium to stop the coagulation
Green stoppered	Either lithium heparin or sodium heparin	Stopping the prothrombin-to-thrombin reaction

FIGURE 1.21   *Anticoagulants that prevent clotting in tubes.*
© Cengage Learning 2013

to go through the clotting process, but the anticoagulant, if properly mixed with the blood, will prevent this from occurring. The methods that the most commonly used tubes incorporate to prevent clotting are listed in Figure 1.21.

What Figure 1.21 illustrates is that the anticoagulants work in a variety of methods to prevent the blood from clotting. This is why one type of tube or the plasma/serum from a tube often cannot be substituted for another. Some examples of problems that can occur when an incorrect sample is sent include the following:

1. A blood sample is collected in a sodium heparin green-stoppered tube, and the plasma is pulled off to test for a sodium level on the patient. The sodium level of the patient will be falsely elevated due to the sodium in the anticoagulant.

2. A blood sample is collected in a gray-stoppered tube and submitted for a CBC. The gray-stoppered tube will not work as a replacement for the lavender-stoppered tube. The EDTA

anticoagulant in the lavender-stoppered tube preserves the morphology of the red blood cells (RBCs) and WBCs. If the gray-stoppered tube is used to determine the CBC results, the cells will appear abnormal and the patient's normal cells could be reported as abnormal.

3. A lavender-stoppered tube is used instead of a clot tube for a calcium test. The person drawing the blood feels no one will notice the mistake and centrifuges the lavender-stoppered tube. The plasma is pulled off and sent to the laboratory. The results indicate that the patient has a zero calcium level. This is a result of the anticoagulant, EDTA, removing the calcium from the plasma to prevent the blood from clotting.

4. A light blue–stoppered tube is used to collect a sample from the patient, and the phlebotomist notices before taking the needle out of the patient's arm that the tube did not fill completely. A second tube is drawn, and it does not fill completely. To submit a completely filled tube as is required, the two half-filled tubes are poured together. The patient's test result will be incorrect because by pouring the two tubes together, the amount of anticoagulant in the combined tube is doubled.

Unfortunately there is no "one size fits all" in the collection of blood samples. The testing methods are very specific and require the correct sample type. A specific tube must be used for a specific test. Anticoagulant tubes that are partially filled should never be poured together to obtain a full tube. This will cause an increased amount of anticoagulant to blood in that tube. Mixing of blood samples from different tubes or combining two half-filled tubes can potentially cause erroneous test results for the patient.

Blood Collection Equipment

All blood collection equipment uses invasive techniques to open a vein to obtain a sample. The common equipment used today punctures the vein and evacuates the blood sample without destroying the integrity of the vein.

The recommended length of the needle used in venipuncture is 1 to 1 1/2 inches. The gauges of needles used are 27, 25, 23, 22, 21, 20, 18, and 16, with the smallest-diameter needle being a 25 gauge and the largest being a 16 gauge.

The needles come in different gauges for the different-size veins that need to be accessed or the amount of blood that needs to be taken. For a child, or an adult when only one tube of blood must be collected, a 23- or 22-gauge needle is appropriate. When someone is donating a unit of blood, the blood needs to be collected faster, so a 16- or 18-gauge needle is used. The needle should be thought of as a pipeline. The faster you want the blood to flow, the larger the pipeline you will need. Consideration must also be made for the size of the vein. The pipeline must fit inside the vein. Therefore, the needle must be small enough to fit inside the vein. This size also partially controls the vacuum of the blood pulling on the vein. A large needle with a large evacuated tube produces a large amount of vacuum on the vein and may possibly collapse the vein. A smaller needle paired with a smaller tube reduces the vacuum.

Needle Gauge	Needle Use
27	Administration of purified protein derivative (PPD) tuberculosis skin test
25	Intramuscular injections
23	Butterfly (winged infusion set) collection system or syringe collection
22	Syringe or evacuated system collection
21	Syringe or evacuated system collection
20	Syringe or evacuated system collection
18	IVs or blood donation
16	IVs or blood donation

The 25-gauge needle cannot be used for venipuncture because the red blood cells would be destroyed (hemolyzed) when blood is pulled through the bore of the needle. The best alternative is to use a 23-gauge needle with a butterfly collection set. This gives access to small veins but does not result in hemolysis of the cells.

Needle size is the choice of the phlebotomist. The phlebotomist must analyze each situation and determine the best equipment to obtain the blood sample.

All needles for venipuncture are manufactured with an angled bevel on the tip of the needle. This bevel helps the needle enter the skin and reduces the pain upon entry. It also gives a larger opening in the tip of the needle to enhance blood flow.

Syringe System

The syringe and needle method of collecting blood is one of the oldest methods known that does not destroy the integrity of the vein. The principle and basic construction have remained the same: a sleeve with a plunger that fits inside, and a needle attached to the other end. The barrel and plunger vary in volume from 1 milliliter to 60 milliliters. The plunger creates a vacuum within the barrel. The plunger on a syringe often sticks and is hard to pull. A technique called "breathing the syringe" needs to be done before it is used. To "breathe" the syringe, pull back on the plunger slightly and then push the plunger back to remove all the air. This makes the plunger pull more smoothly and reduces the tendency to jerk when first pulled.

A large syringe collects more blood, but it can also create a problem, producing too much vacuum and collapsing the vein. Pulling the plunger slowly and resting between pulls allows the vein time to refill with blood and prevents collapse of the vein. Generally syringes are used for the difficult-to-draw patients who have fragile, thin, or "rolly" veins. Pediatric or geriatric patients typically have these types of veins. The use of a syringe and needle is limited by the capacity of the syringe. The use of a syringe larger than 10 to 15 milliliters to collect blood from fragile veins is not recommended. If a large amount of blood is needed, a butterfly collection set is to be used. Syringes are

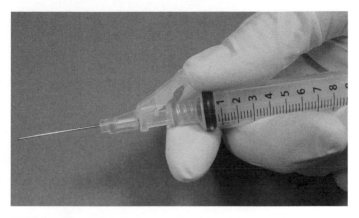

FIGURE 1.22 *Syringe and needle with safety sleeve for needle.*
© Cengage Learning 2013

also used in special procedures when the blood must be drawn and then transferred to a different container.

For the protection of the phlebotomist, the syringe should have a safety shield that covers the needle incorporated into the device (Figure 1.22).

Evacuated System

The evacuated system is often called the Vacutainer system. Vacutainer can be a misnomer, because it is a brand name for the evacuated system manufactured by the Becton Dickinson Company. The Vacutainer name has become synonymous with all evacuated blood collection systems.

The evacuated blood collection system is a closed system that adds an element of safety. In the evacuated system, a tube containing a vacuum attaches to the needle and the tube's vacuum is replaced by blood. The tubes can be glass or plastic (Figure 1.23). The total system consists of a double-pointed needle, a plastic holder or adapter, and a series of vacuum tubes with rubber stoppers. One end of the double-pointed needle enters the patient, and the opposite end of the needle punctures the stopper of the tube.

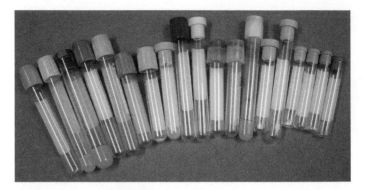

FIGURE 1.23 *Assorted types of evacuated tubes.*
© Cengage Learning 2013

The key to the evacuated system is the double-pointed needle with a different-length needle on each end and a screw hub near the center. The longer needle has a bevel that enters the vein. The shorter needle pierces the rubber stopper in the blood collection tube. The needle that pierces the rubber stopper of the tube has a sleeve that functions as a valve to stop the flow of blood when the tube is removed. Pushing the tube into the holder compresses the sleeve and exposes the needle as it enters the tube. When removing the tube, the sleeve slides back over the needle and stops the flow of blood.

The needles are manufactured in two configurations. The basic needle is straight with no safety devices attached. Use of this needle requires the safety shield to be attached to the holder. The alternate needle has the safety device attached to the needle (Figure 1.24).

The needle is a pipeline that is going to deliver blood from the patient to the tube. The blood is pulled out of the patient due to the vacuum inside the tube. The patient will experience the least pain if the bevel of the needle is facing upward when inserted into the vein. The bevel of the needle is upward when looking straight down on the needle as the needle is inserted into the skin and the opening in the needle is visible. This technique allows the point of the needle

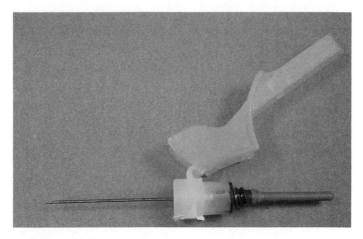

FIGURE 1.24   *Evacuated tube needle with safety shield.*
© Cengage Learning 2013

to enter the skin first with little dragging or bunching up of the skin and reduces the pain of the puncture. To obtain the maximum blood flow, the needle should be inserted at a 15- to 30-degree angle to the surface of the skin (Figure 1.25). The deeper the vein, the greater the angle you will need to use. A shallow vein will be accessed at a 15-degree angle, while a deep vein will need a 30-degree angle for the best entry. Entering at an angle less than or greater than 15 to 30 degrees will increase the chance of missing the vein or causing nerve damage.

The holder for the needle makes the task of collecting the blood sample easier. The holders have changed in recent years to include holders with covers that snap closed over the contaminated needle (Figure 1.26).

Butterfly (Winged Infusion Set) Collection System

A winged infusion set (butterfly) consists of a 1/2- to 3/4-inch stainless steel needle connected to a 6- to 12-inch length of tubing. It is called a butterfly because of its wing-shaped plastic extensions, which are used

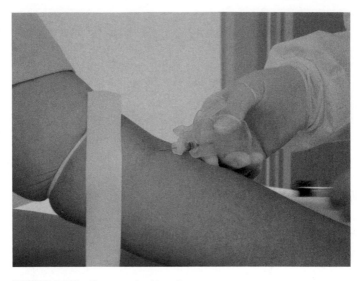

FIGURE 1.25   *Proper angle of insertion.*
© Cengage Learning 2013

for gripping the needle. Butterfly needles for venipuncture are 25, 23, or 21 gauge. A 25-gauge butterfly and syringe should be avoided because of an increased chance for hemolysis. The needle should have a safety device in order to meet Occupational Safety and Health Administration (OSHA) requirements. This device generally consists of a sleeve that slides over the needle immediately after use or a needle that retracts from the patient's arm.

Butterflies generally come with ports that allow them to be used with syringes or with multiple sample Leur adapters, allowing them to be used with an evacuated tube system. Leur adapters are also available singly to convert the port of a butterfly for use with the evacuated tube system.

The butterfly system is for small veins that are difficult to draw with the evacuated tube system and standard evacuated tube system needle. The winged needle of the butterfly slides into a small surface vein. Instead of entering the vein at the usual 15-degree angle, the winged

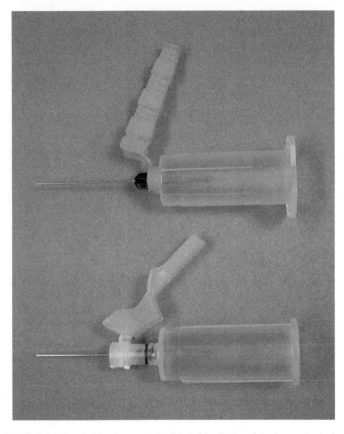

FIGURE 1.26   *Safety sleeve attached to holder (top); safety sleeve attached to needle (bottom).*
© Cengage Learning 2013

needle is inserted at approximately a 5-degree angle and then threaded into the vein. This procedure anchors the needle in the center of even a small vein. If the patient moves, the tubing gives flexibility so the needle will stay anchored and not pull out of the vein. The butterfly collection set works well on children and adults who have both small veins and the tendency to move while blood is being collected. The tubing also works as a pressure relief valve. An evacuated tube or syringe can be attached to the tubing and the vein will not collapse, as would normally occur. Drawing blood too quickly with a syringe will collapse the vein.

The butterfly system also provides the adaptability of initiating a draw with a syringe and then finishing it with the evacuated tube system. A syringe can be used for procedures that require a syringe sample, which is then removed and the evacuated tube system attached for multiple tube collection. Although the butterfly collection system has many benefits, it is not used for all collection. It is much more expensive than the needle system. The additional expense is unnecessary for the majority of venipunctures. Butterfly needles should be used only 10 to 15 percent of the time on the average adult patient. This percentage will be greater in pediatric hospitals and oncology centers where the patients' veins require the use of a smaller needle.

Needle Safety

The Needlestick Safety and Prevention Act revised OSHA's blood-borne pathogen standard. There are several parts to this law, but the part affecting the phlebotomist is the portion that addresses "changes in technology that eliminate or reduce exposure to bloodborne pathogens." For the phlebotomist this means switching to what are known as "needlestick prevention devices." There are multiple devices on the market to be used with whatever type of needle is used. Figure 1.22 shows a safety sleeve that slides over the syringe needle. Figure 1.24 shows the safety sleeve attached to the needle and pushed by the thumb. Other devices attach to the holder instead of the needle. The locking cover protects the phlebotomist from needlesticks until the needle and holder can be discarded into a puncture-proof sharps container. Examples of butterfly safety devices are shown in Figure 1.27.

After use, the needle must remain attached to the holder and the entire needle and holder assembly must be discarded into a sharps

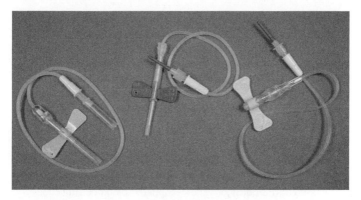

FIGURE 1.27 *Butterfly needles for use with evacuated system.*
© Cengage Learning 2013

container. The reason for not removing the needle is to avoid exposure of the part of the needle that punctures the tube. By not removing the needle from the holder, that end of the needle is shielded by the holder to prevent accidental needlestick.

Cleaning of the Draw Site

Antiseptics are used to clean the skin surface before a venipuncture, capillary puncture, or arterial puncture. Antiseptics are chemical solutions that reduce the number of bacteria on the skin surface. Work practice controls dictate that to prevent infection of the patients or the health care worker, antiseptic solutions must be used. Types of antiseptics available include the following:

- 70 percent isopropyl alcohol either saturated into gauze or in prepackaged pads.

- Tincture of iodine or povidone-iodine. These come as pads or swabs and are mostly used for skin prep for blood cultures or arterial punctures.

- 2 percent chlorhexidine gluconate and 70 percent isopropyl alcohol, used for skin prep for blood cultures.

- Benzalkonium chloride, an alternate skin cleanser.
- Zephrin chloride, an alternate skin cleanser.
- Hydrogen peroxide, an alternate when there are allergies to alcohol.

Order of Drawing Tubes

With multiple draws using the evacuated system, the order of drawing the tubes is important. The recommended order of draw for direct collection into an evacuated system is as follows:

1. Blood culture bottle or yellow-stoppered blood culture tube (sterile procedure)
2. Coagulation tube (e.g., light-blue stoppered)
3. Serum tube with or without clot activator or gel serum separator (e.g., red stoppered, red/black stoppered, plastic or glass)
4. Heparin tube with or without gel plasma separator (e.g., green stoppered)
5. EDTA tube (e.g., lavender stoppered)
6. Oxalate/fluoride, glycolytic inhibitor tube (e.g., gray stoppered)

If not all the tubes in the order of draw are to be collected, the order is started with the first tube needing collection. If all that needs to be collected is a green-stoppered tube and a lavender-stoppered tube, the green-stoppered tube is collected first, followed by the lavender-stoppered tube.

With requests for routine coagulation testing, such as PT and aPTT, that use a light blue–stoppered tube, the first tube collected can still be the light blue–stoppered tube.

There are two exceptions to this. When a butterfly is used, there is air in the tubing of the butterfly. For a light blue–stoppered tube that must be completely full to maintain the 1:9 anticoagulant-to-blood ratio, the air in the tubing will reduce the amount of blood in the tube. Therefore, a plain-stoppered tube (no clot activator) or a light blue–stoppered tube must be drawn as a discard tube first to clear the air from the tubing. A second exception when a discard tube is collected

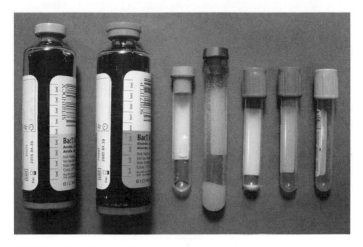

FIGURE 1.28   *Tubes in the correct order of draw.*
© Cengage Learning 2013

first is with special coagulation testing. For special coagulation testing (factor assays), a plain red-stoppered tube (no clot activator) or a light blue–stoppered tube must be drawn as a discard tube first. This clears the draw site of a clotting substance called thromboplastin that is produced by the body as a result of the puncture.

The reasoning for an order of draw is that sterile collection tubes are collected first to prevent bacterial contamination. The anticoagulant tubes are drawn in the order indicated to avoid cross contamination of the anticoagulants. As a tube is pulled out of the evacuated tube holder, the needle is coated with a small amount of anticoagulant. This anticoagulant is then injected into the next tube drawn. If the heparin tube were drawn before the citrate tube, the citrate tube would have a small amount of heparin added to it and the patient's coagulation test results would appear as if the patient was on a blood thinner. An EDTA tube drawn before the green-stoppered tube can give a falsely elevated potassium.

Figure 1.28 shows the tubes in the correct order of draw.

UNIT 2
VENIPUNCTURE TECHNIQUE

Sample Labeling

*P*roper patient identification and sample labeling are as simple as drawing the correct patient's blood and labeling it with the correct name. All patient samples must be positively identified on the primary container to avoid any errors in reporting of results, thereby affecting patient diagnosis or treatment. Improper patient identification and sample labeling are the most common sources of error in phlebotomy. These errors can be easily avoided by following the simple steps shown in Procedure 2.1.

PROCEDURE 2.1 Proper Patient and Sample Identification

Principle:

To verify patient identification prior to sample collection.

Procedure:

1. All requests for laboratory testing must have a requisition or computer labels. The requisition must include the patient's first and last names, test(s) requested, diagnosis, and name of ordering physician.

2. Every associate collecting a sample from a patient checks two verifiers to ensure correct patient identification. Approach the patient in a professional and courteous manner. The patient will be unsure of what you are going to do. Explain the process you are going to perform and remember to focus on the patient and ignore outside distractions.

   a. Reading from the requisition or label, call the patient using the full name on the requisition or label.

   b. Before drawing the sample, ask the patient to spell his or her last name and state the date of birth using the requisition as verification. A patient whose sample is to be drawn for any blood bank procedure must be identified by an additional means besides the preceding procedure if he or she is

continues

PROCEDURE 2.1 Proper Patient and Sample Identification *continued*

an outpatient. The preferred identification sources for outpatients are as follows:

   i. A driver's license with a current address

   ii. If the address is not current, then a driver's license and a personal check with the current address

   iii. Another form of identification with a current address

c. If the patient is unable to verbally provide the information, a parent/guardian, nurse, or current picture ID may be used.

d. Computer-generated labels should be verified with the requisition for correct name before collecting the sample.

3. After ensuring that you have the correct patient, perform the venipuncture.

4. The tube(s) are labeled by the individual obtaining the sample before leaving the patient.

a. The following must be included on the label:

   i. Patient's name (no nicknames)

   ii. Medical record number, if available

   iii. Patient's birth date (for blood bank testing)

   iv. Date and time collected

continues

PROCEDURE 2.1 Proper Patient and Sample Identification *continued*

      v. Source of the sample (if other than blood)

     vi. Initials of individual obtaining the sample

   b. Aliquots or dilutions must be labeled with the following:

      i. Patient's name (no nicknames)

     ii. Collection date and time

    iii. Type of sample (plasma, serum, etc.)

   c. Timed collections must also be labeled with the time of collection and the type of collection (e.g., pre-, post-, fasting, 1 hour, 2 hour).

5. Read each label as it is attached to the tube before leaving the patient. Compare one label to another to ensure that all labels are for this patient.

6. If computer labels are unavailable, labeling of the tubes may be done by (a) imprinted labels or (b) handwriting the patient's complete first and last names, hospital registration number(s), room number, date and time of draw as required by the test, and phlebotomist's initials.

7. If the patient does not have an identification band on his or her wrist or ankle, or if the identification band is not correct, notify the nurse or nursing unit secretary. Do not draw blood unless the patient is wearing a correct identification band.

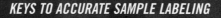

KEYS TO ACCURATE SAMPLE LABELING

1. Sample tubes should not be prelabeled.
2. Take laboratory labels to the bedside or outpatient location or handwrite labels at the patient's side.
3. Compare each label to the others to verify that they are all for the same patient.
4. Compare the labels to the patient to verify that you are ready to draw a sample from the correct patient.
5. Label all filled tubes BEFORE YOU LEAVE THE PATIENT. Tubes are to be labeled by the person doing the collecting.
6. Note the date and time for each sample collected.
7. Initial all tubes to verify all information on patient identification is correct.
8. Write the test name on the label.
9. Do not place unlabeled samples in emesis basins, cups, or bags and label the container. If a sample is held for possible testing later, it should be properly labeled and initialed by the associate who did the collection.
10. Labeled samples are then bagged and sent to the proper laboratory.

Computer systems are replacing many of the manual requisitions. Hospitals now use computer systems consistently and only use manual systems when the computer system is down. Outpatient laboratory service centers also use computers to hold patient information for patients who return to the center and to print labels. This helps the laboratory and the patient by having addresses and billing information

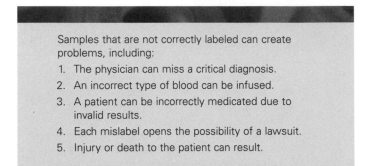

Samples that are not correctly labeled can create problems, including:
1. The physician can miss a critical diagnosis.
2. An incorrect type of blood can be infused.
3. A patient can be incorrectly medicated due to invalid results.
4. Each mislabel opens the possibility of a lawsuit.
5. Injury or death to the patient can result.

readily available. Some laboratory computer systems are linked to the physician's office, so that the physician can order tests in the office and then have the patient go to the outpatient center to obtain the sample. When the patient arrives, the laboratory is able to access the orders, collect the sample, and send the sample to the testing laboratory. When the testing is completed, the physician can look up the patient's results wherever there is computer access.

Inaccuracy in patient identification and sample labeling can cause serious problems for the patient.

Test Request Form

A test request form lists the information needed for the phlebotomist to complete the task. The patient's physician initiates the test request form. The following information should be included on the form:

- Patient's complete name and age or date of birth
- Patient identification number
- Date and time sample is to be obtained
- Type of test to be collected
- Accessioning number

- Physician's name
- Department or location where the work is to be done (on computer requests)
- Other information necessary to accurately collect the sample, such as specific time of collection, fasting, and so forth
- ICD-9 diagnosis codes for outpatients

Precautions in Blood Collection

Phlebotomists must be aware of various concerns that affect them or the outcome of the testing on a patient. Some of these are the result of procedural inconsistencies by the phlebotomist, whereas others are caused by the health of the patient. A few, as with latex allergies, can affect the health of the phlebotomist or the patient.

Hemoconcentration

Hemoconcentration is the increased concentration of constituents in the blood resulting from the tourniquet being left on too long. The tourniquet should not be left on the arm longer than 1 minute. If the tourniquet has restricted blood flow for longer than 1 minute the laboratory test results will possibly be invalid. This occurs because of a decrease in blood volume from fluid moving from the veins into the tissue. Those analytes that are too large to pass through the vascular wall are concentrated in the blood. Analytes such as calcium, cholesterol, lipids, drugs, steroids, and thyroid hormones increase.

To prevent hemoconcentration, do not leave the tourniquet on longer than 1 minute before venipuncture. If it takes longer than 1 minute to select a vein, remove the tourniquet for 2 minutes, then reapply the tourniquet.

Hematoma

A leakage of blood out of the vein during or after venipuncture causes a hematoma. A bruise will result. At the first sign of a hematoma the phlebotomist should discontinue the venipuncture and apply heavy pressure to the site. This accumulation of blood under the skin produces a discoloration on the skin, and the pressure of the buildup of blood can cause pain in the arm of the patient.

The following steps can help prevent a hematoma:

1. Remove the tourniquet before removing the needle.
2. Apply a small amount of pressure to the area after removal of the needle. Also tightly apply an adhesive bandage over the gauze.
3. Do not use superficial veins.
4. Puncture only the uppermost wall of the vein. Do not puncture through both sides of the vein.
5. Make sure the needle fully punctures the uppermost wall of the vein. Partial penetration may allow the blood to leak into the tissue surrounding the vein.

Hemolysis

Hemolysis is the breaking or rupturing of the membrane of the red blood cells. Contents of the red blood cells then "contaminate" the serum or plasma to be tested. The serum or plasma appears slightly pink to a clear red in color. The laboratory tests are therefore inaccurate. Potassium is the first element to be affected.

The following steps can help prevent hemolysis:

1. Do not draw from a hematoma or bruised area.
2. Avoid using too small a needle, such as a 25 gauge.
3. Avoid drawing back the plunger of a syringe too forcefully.
4. Avoid foaming or frothing of the blood as it enters the syringe.
5. Let the alcohol on the puncture site air dry before inserting the needle.

Icteric Blood

Icteric blood, which results when a patient's serum or plasma contains a large amount of bilirubin because of jaundice, is blood that has a yellow to orange color. The patient's skin and the sclera of the eyes may also have the same yellow to orange color. This is caused by the patient's condition and not a blood collection error.

Lipemic Blood

Blood is lipemic when a large amount of fats and lipids are present in the blood, giving the serum and the plasma a white, milky color. This type of serum or plasma is known as lipemic. This is the result of the patient's condition and not a blood collection error.

Intravenous Line

Intravenous (IV) lines supply needed fluids and medicines to the patient. When an intravenous solution is being administered into one arm, blood should not be drawn from that arm. Blood drawn from the arm containing the IV solution has the potential to contaminate the blood sample. IV lines are inserted into a vein. The site can be anywhere from the back of the hand to farther up the arm. IV sites are generally not placed in the upper area of the arm but in any site below the upper arm. That makes the upper arm area very tempting to draw blood from because the veins can be felt in the upper arm and the IV is in the lower part of the arm. Venous blood is flowing up the arm from the hand to the shoulder. The IV solution is flowing in that direction. Any blood drawn in a site above the IV will contain the IV solution. The IV solution will be in a high concentration because it has not had a chance to circulate through the body. As a result, the laboratory test results will be higher or lower depending on the contents of the IV solution.

To avoid this kind of error, the phlebotomist should look for a blood-drawing site in the opposite arm. Occasionally, an IV is running in both arms and no site can be found except in the area of the IV. Satisfactory samples can be drawn below the IV (never above) by following several precautions. Preferably have the IV shut off for at least 2 minutes before venipuncture. (The phlebotomist must never shut off a running IV. The nurse or physician of that patient must make the decision to shut off an IV, even temporarily.) Apply the tourniquet below the IV site. Select a vein other than the one with the IV. Perform the venipuncture. Draw 7 to 10 milliliters of blood and discard this blood to clear any IV solutions from the arm before test samples are collected.

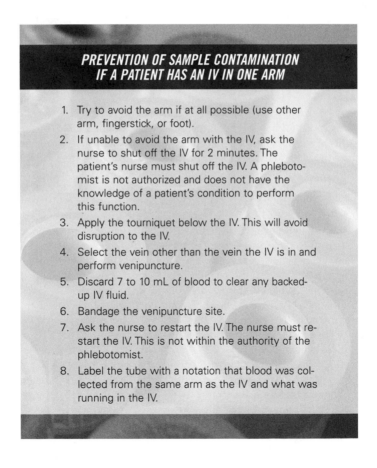

PREVENTION OF SAMPLE CONTAMINATION IF A PATIENT HAS AN IV IN ONE ARM

1. Try to avoid the arm if at all possible (use other arm, fingerstick, or foot).
2. If unable to avoid the arm with the IV, ask the nurse to shut off the IV for 2 minutes. The patient's nurse must shut off the IV. A phlebotomist is not authorized and does not have the knowledge of a patient's condition to perform this function.
3. Apply the tourniquet below the IV. This will avoid disruption to the IV.
4. Select the vein other than the vein the IV is in and perform venipuncture.
5. Discard 7 to 10 mL of blood to clear any backed-up IV fluid.
6. Bandage the venipuncture site.
7. Ask the nurse to restart the IV. The nurse must restart the IV. This is not within the authority of the phlebotomist.
8. Label the tube with a notation that blood was collected from the same arm as the IV and what was running in the IV.

Vascular Access Device (Line)

A vascular access device (VAD), also called an indwelling line or heparin/saline well, consists of tubing inserted into a main vein or artery (Figure 2.1). It is used primarily for administering fluids and medications, monitoring pressures, and drawing blood. Specially trained individuals should be the only persons with VAD access. Because lines are routinely flushed with heparin or saline, a discard volume of blood must be drawn. For adults, a discard volume of 7 to 10 milliliters is drawn. If the proper discard volume is not drawn, the laboratory test results will be erroneous.

This procedure is generally reserved for the nurse or physician of the patient and cannot be completed by the phlebotomist.

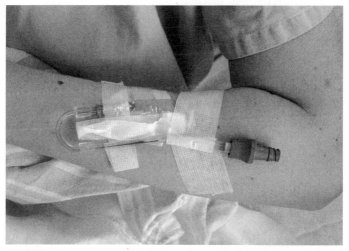

FIGURE 2.1   *Heparin/saline well.*
© Cengage Learning 2013

Handwashing

Handwashing is the single most important means of preventing the spread of infection. Hands must be washed under running water with soap and vigorous rubbing. When the soap is rinsed off, the water should flow from the wrists to the fingertips. See Procedure 1.1 for proper handwashing technique. Alcohol-based hand cleaners are acceptable in place of handwashing. The hand cleaners have become widely accepted because even when running water is available, people are more likely to use hand cleaner than to wash hands. It is very simple, when going from one patient to another, to rub hand cleaner into your hands. This takes less time than a proper handwashing. Because most people do not spend sufficient time washing their hands, the hand cleaner does a more thorough job. Handwashing with soap and water must be done if there is visible blood on the hands.

Latex Allergy

Latex, which is made from the natural rubber of trees, can be found in many household and health care products. Balloons, toys, garden hoses, rubber gloves, tourniquets, IV tubing, blood pressure cuffs, and bandages are a few of the products that can contain latex. Allergies to latex have been on the increase because there is more exposure to latex products. Phlebotomists are at high risk due to their constant exposure to latex tourniquets and latex gloves. Patients are also showing an increased sensitivity to latex due to environmental exposure. Signs should be placed for the patient to remind the health care worker of his or her latex allergy.

Reactions to latex can vary with the individual, from itchy irritation to redness and swelling, progressing to thickened skin, pimples, or skin blisters that ooze. This is the typical, less serious type IV allergy to latex due to irritant contact dermatitis. Symptoms begin 24 to 72 hours after exposure and can continue for several days. With each additional exposure, the symptoms become more advanced. For some patients, the latex allergy becomes so severe that they cannot go into a room where latex items have been used.

Type I latex allergy is more serious. This is an immunological reaction that is caused by the penetration of the natural latex proteins into the skin. These proteins cause a production of antibodies to latex that increases with each subsequent exposure. As the allergy becomes more severe, the symptoms may include nausea, low blood pressure, and respiratory distress. If the latex allergen is introduced directly into the blood, anaphylactic shock is possible. This can be life threatening.

To prevent allergic reactions, exposure to latex must be eliminated. There is no cure for latex allergy, only prevention of exposure. This prevention of exposure is not only for the phlebotomist but also for the patient. If the phlebotomist has a latex allergy, latex gloves or tourniquets must not be used. If the patient has a latex allergy, the phlebotomist must avoid any type of latex contact to the patient. This includes the tourniquet, latex gloves, blood pressure cuffs, and adhesive bandages.

Latex allergies do not always come in the form of direct contact to the skin. The powder in the gloves disperses the latex into the air, and then the phlebotomist or the patient inhales the powder, producing a respiratory reaction. A less serious form of powder allergy occurs when powder gets in the eyes and the eyes become irritated and swollen. Most health care providers are switching to latex-free, powder-free gloves to avoid problems.

Collecting the Venipuncture Blood Sample

Positioning the Patient

The position of the patient is critical for proper patient blood collection. The best position is one that is comfortable for the patient and the phlebotomist. Proper positioning of the patient makes the patient feel more at ease, and the phlebotomist is better able to perform the venipuncture. In most critical care situations the patient is reclining, the ideal position to draw blood. If the patient is ambulatory, then proper patient position must be maintained.

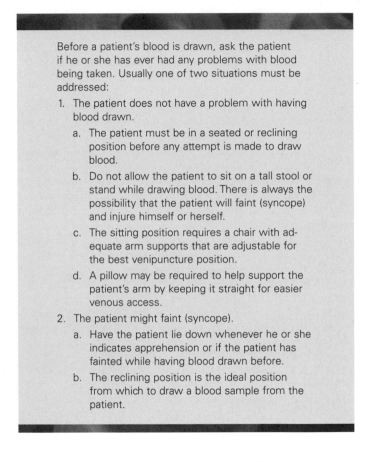

Before a patient's blood is drawn, ask the patient if he or she has ever had any problems with blood being taken. Usually one of two situations must be addressed:

1. The patient does not have a problem with having blood drawn.

   a. The patient must be in a seated or reclining position before any attempt is made to draw blood.

   b. Do not allow the patient to sit on a tall stool or stand while drawing blood. There is always the possibility that the patient will faint (syncope) and injure himself or herself.

   c. The sitting position requires a chair with adequate arm supports that are adjustable for the best venipuncture position.

   d. A pillow may be required to help support the patient's arm by keeping it straight for easier venous access.

2. The patient might faint (syncope).

   a. Have the patient lie down whenever he or she indicates apprehension or if the patient has fainted while having blood drawn before.

   b. The reclining position is the ideal position from which to draw a blood sample from the patient.

Selecting the Appropriate Venipuncture Site

The appropriate venipuncture site can vary depending on the patient. The usual site that is first checked is the upper bend of the arm (antecubital fossa). The primary vein used in the upper arm is the median cubital vein. This is usually the prominent vein in the middle of the bend of the arm (Figure 2.2).

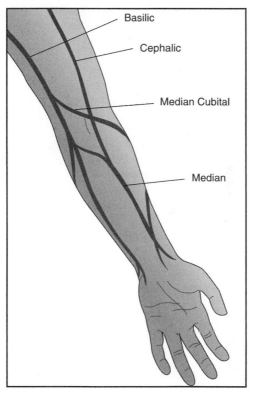

FIGURE 2.2 *Superficial veins in the arm.*
© Cengage Learning 2013

The basilic, cephalic, or median veins can be used as an alternative. After the median cubital vein, the cephalic vein is the next preferred site. The basilic vein is the least preferred because along this vein is the brachial artery and major nerves. When attempting a venipuncture in the area of the basilic vein you must be careful to not go too deep to avoid damage to the brachial artery or nerve. If these veins are not accessible or not prominent enough to obtain a blood sample from, go to the back of the hand to determine other possibilities. The veins in the back of the hand have the tendency to "roll" more than the arm veins because they are not supported by as much tissue and they are closer to the surface. To avoid this, the vein must be held in place below the puncture site with your thumb while a smaller-gauge needle or a butterfly is used. The hand veins are best accessed with a 3- to 5-milliliter syringe with a 22-gauge needle or a 23-gauge butterfly (winged infusion set). The wrist veins are also an alternative but generally are much more painful than the other sites. The wrist vein that is accessible is the vein that is in line with the thumb. By following the thumb up to the wrist area, a predominant vein on top of the wrist is usually found. The foot and ankle veins may also be used only if the patient's physician gives permission. The veins in the foot or ankle also have the tendency to roll.

Only two attempts should be made to draw from a patient. If all the alternatives have failed to reveal an acceptable venipuncture site, then a more experienced phlebotomist should check. If venous access is not possible, determine if it is possible to collect the sample from a fingerstick.

Vein Stimulation

The tourniquet makes the veins more prominent by restricting the venous flow and inhibiting the arterial flow of blood in the arm. The tourniquet is a soft, pliable, rubber strip approximately 1 inch wide by

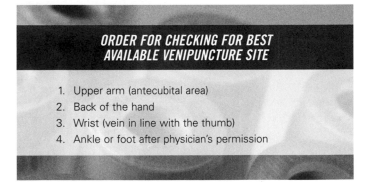

ORDER FOR CHECKING FOR BEST AVAILABLE VENIPUNCTURE SITE

1. Upper arm (antecubital area)
2. Back of the hand
3. Wrist (vein in line with the thumb)
4. Ankle or foot after physician's permission

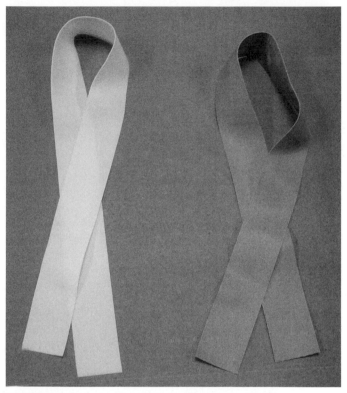

FIGURE 2.3 *Latex tourniquet (left), nonlatex tourniquet (right).*
© Cengage Learning 2013

15 to 18 inches long. The tourniquet can be either latex or nonlatex for patients or phlebotomists with latex allergies (Figure 2.3).

The strip tourniquet is best for all conditions. The rubber strip can easily be released with one hand. Because it is about 1 inch wide, it does not cut into the patient's arm but distributes the pressure. Tourniquets are inexpensive enough that they can be discarded after each use. When tying a tourniquet, the ends should be pointed upward to prevent the ends from falling down on the venipuncture site.

Procedure 2.2 outlines the procedure for tying and releasing a tourniquet.

PROCEDURE 2.2 Tying and Releasing a Tourniquet

Principle:
To properly tie a tourniquet to constrict blood flow for venous access but not compromise circulation.

Procedure:

1. Determine if you can use a latex tourniquet or if you will need a nonlatex tourniquet. Preferably always use a nonlatex tourniquet.

2. Inspect the patient's arms for the most likely vein to use.

3. Wrap the tourniquet around the arm 3 to 4 inches above the likely venipuncture site. Keep the tourniquet flat to minimize the discomfort to the patient (Figure 2.4).

4. Stretch the tourniquet, bring both ends to the front of the patient, and cross the ends of the tourniquet (Figure 2.5).

5. While holding the ends tight, tuck one portion of the tourniquet under the other. This is usually the end of the tourniquet that is the lower of the two (nearest the hand) (Figure 2.6).

6. By tucking the lower of the two ends, the loose ends of the tourniquet are facing upward and should not be a hindrance to the venipuncture (Figure 2.7).

continues

PROCEDURE 2.2 Tying and Releasing a Tourniquet
continued

7. The tourniquet should now cause the veins to be more prominent.

8. To release the tourniquet, pull on the end of the tourniquet that you tucked.

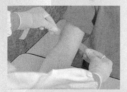

FIGURE 2.4 *Wrap the tourniquet around the arm 3 to 4 inches above the likely venipuncture site. Keep the tourniquet flat to minimize the discomfort to the patient.*

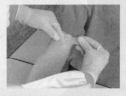

FIGURE 2.5 *Stretch the tourniquet and bring both ends to the front of the patient and cross the ends of the tourniquet.*

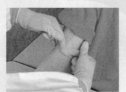

FIGURE 2.6 *While holding the ends tight, tuck one portion of the tourniquet under the other.*

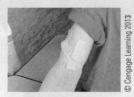

FIGURE 2.7 *By tucking the lower of the two ends, the loose ends of the tourniquet are facing upward and are not a hindrance to the venipuncture.*

© Cengage Learning 2013

A tourniquet must be used to assist the phlebotomist in feeling a vein. The tourniquet is applied 3 to 4 inches above the puncture site. It is applied tightly enough to slow the flow of blood in the veins but not so tightly as to prevent the flow of blood in the arteries. This is similar to damming a small stream. When the stream is dammed, the water forms a pond behind the dam. With the tourniquet applied, the veins fill with blood, pooling in the veins below the tourniquet. This pooling of blood makes the veins more prominent. The vein must be palpated with the tip of the index finger to determine its depth and size. Feel for and trace the path of the vein several times. Avoid using the thumb because it has a pulse and is not as sensitive as the rest of the fingers. The vein feels soft and bouncy to the touch. The roundness of the vein and the direction it follows may be determined. All veins are not straight up and down the arm. If no veins become prominent, retie the tourniquet tighter but not so tightly as to stop the flow of arterial blood into the arm. If the tourniquet is tied tightly enough to stop arterial blood flow, the patient will no longer have a pulse in the wrist. If this occurs, immediately remove the tourniquet, because this indicates that blood has ceased below the tourniquet. If a vein cannot be felt, several methods may be used to stimulate vein prominence (see Methods of Vein Stimulation).

The tourniquet often causes greater discomfort for patients than the venipuncture itself. Ideally the tourniquet should be removed as soon as

METHODS OF VEIN STIMULATION

1. Position the arm lower than the patient.
2. Reapply the tourniquet.
3. Massage the arm in an upward motion.
4. Use a blood pressure cuff in place of the tourniquet.
5. Warm the venipuncture site with a warming device or a warm washcloth.

blood flow is established. The act of removing the tourniquet may move the needle or vein just enough so that no more blood can be obtained and a second venipuncture must be performed. It is recommended to wait until just before the needle is removed from the patient to remove the tourniquet. If the tourniquet is not removed before the needle is removed, the patient will bleed heavily. Blood will be forced out of the needle hole and into the surrounding tissue, resulting in a hematoma.

There are several situations in which venipuncture should be avoided (Figure 2.8). If the "vein" that is felt has a pulsing action to

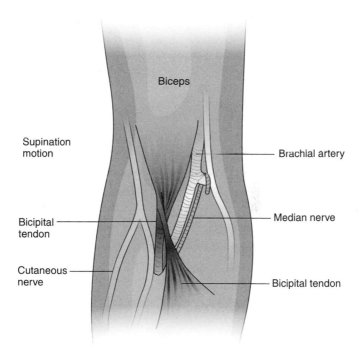

FIGURE 2.8 *Venipuncture sites to avoid.*
© Cengage Learning 2013

it, this indicates that it is an artery, not a vein, and the vessel should not be punctured. Tendons can be deceptive and give the appearance of a vein. They do not have the soft, bouncy feel and are hard to the touch. Puncturing a tendon gives no blood return and is painful to the patient. There are also nerves that run the length of the arm. The nerves cannot be seen or felt, but by avoiding deep, probing venipunctures, the chance of touching a nerve is diminished. If the patient complains that the venipuncture is extremely painful, immediately stop and try another site.

In a patient who has edematous arms that are swollen due to fluid in the tissue, the veins will not be prominent and the tourniquet will not be effective because of the swelling of the arm. Using the tourniquet leaves a temporary indentation in the arm and has the potential to cause tissue damage. Areas of scarring should also be avoided due to possible injury or excessive pain to the patient. Samples collected from an area of a hematoma may produce erroneous test results. If another vein site is not available, the sample is collected distal from the hematoma. Arms with fistulas should also be avoided. Because of the potential for harm to the patient due to lymphostasis, the arm on

VENIPUNCTURE SITES TO AVOID

1. Above an IV site
2. Pulsating arterial areas
3. Tendons or veins without a soft bounce
4. Nerves
5. Edematous areas
6. Side of a mastectomy
7. Cannulas
8. Fistulas
9. Areas of scarring

the side of a mastectomy should be avoided. If the patient has had a double mastectomy, a physician should be consulted prior to drawing the blood. Generally the physician will instruct the phlebotomist to draw from the side of the oldest mastectomy.

Syringe Sample Collection

The patient has been identified, paperwork and tubes have been verified, and equipment has been assembled, and the patient is in a comfortable position. The next step is to tie the tourniquet. Have the patient close the hand, and then select a vein. If possible, place the patient's arm in a downward position. After locating an acceptable vein, mentally map the location. Set mental sights on the vein by visualizing the puncture site as the target. It might be slightly over from this freckle and a little down from that wrinkle. Set those mental sights for an accurate puncture. Cleanse the site with a gauze pad wet with 70 percent isopropyl alcohol solution. A commercially prepared alcohol pad or one with 0.5 percent chlorhexidine in alcohol may also be used. The skin is cleansed in a circular motion from the center to the outside. The area is allowed to air dry to prevent hemolysis of the sample and to prevent the patient from feeling a burning sensation during blood collection.

Some authorities suggest donning gloves first and then palpating for the vein. This technique is required for the patient who is isolated due to a communicable disease and is good practice for all patients. Standard precautions require that personal protective equipment be worn when there is a chance of coming in contact with blood and body fluid. If the patient has veins that are difficult to palpate, gloves may be donned after the site has been palpated and before the cleansing. To avoid forgetting the best location of the collection site, palpate the vein 1 to 2 inches above and below the intended puncture site. It helps the phlebotomist feel that the vein is located in a straight line, and these points can be used to "reset" the mental crosshairs without contaminating the venipuncture site. Goggles and a mask must be worn if there is a potential for blood spatter.

The syringe technique is used less often than the evacuated system. The techniques developed in the syringe method are building blocks for the evacuated tube technique and all other techniques that the phlebotomist uses for obtaining a blood sample.

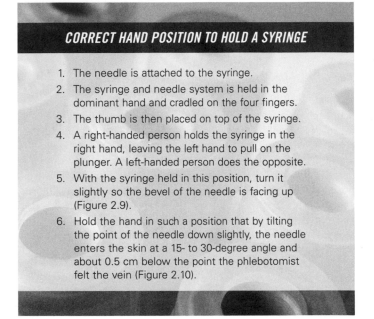

CORRECT HAND POSITION TO HOLD A SYRINGE

1. The needle is attached to the syringe.
2. The syringe and needle system is held in the dominant hand and cradled on the four fingers.
3. The thumb is then placed on top of the syringe.
4. A right-handed person holds the syringe in the right hand, leaving the left hand to pull on the plunger. A left-handed person does the opposite.
5. With the syringe held in this position, turn it slightly so the bevel of the needle is facing up (Figure 2.9).
6. Hold the hand in such a position that by tilting the point of the needle down slightly, the needle enters the skin at a 15- to 30-degree angle and about 0.5 cm below the point the phlebotomist felt the vein (Figure 2.10).

The syringe is ideal for small blood samples in fragile surface veins such as veins in the back of the hand. Procedure 2.3 explains venipuncture with a syringe.

When a syringe is used, the blood obtained must be placed in appropriate containers. Aliquot the blood into evacuated tubes according to step 25 of Procedure 2.3. The preferred method of placing the blood into the evacuated tube is to use a transfer device. This device is similar to an evacuated tube holder except that a syringe can lock into the end of the holder and an evacuated tube can be slid into the holder to accept the blood. The blood is collected with a syringe. The needle's safety mechanism is then activated. Remove the blood-filled syringe from the activated safety needle. Once the needle is removed, the transfer device can be attached to the syringe of blood.

An alternate method is not as safe and does not meet safety standards. It should only be used when there is no transfer device

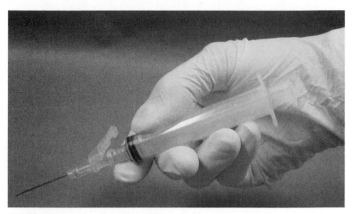

FIGURE 2.9 *Correct hand position to hold a syringe.*
© Cengage Learning 2013

immediately available and the sample will clot before a transfer device can be located. Collect the blood with a syringe and after collection activate the safety shield on the needle. This needle is then removed and a new needle attached once the phlebotomist is at the location where the blood is to be transferred to the evacuated tube. Place the selected tubes to be filled into a test tube rack. Puncture the stopper of the selected tubes with the syringe needle and allow the blood to enter the tube as a result of the tube vacuum. Do not hold the tube to support it; allow the test tube rack to support the tube. If the tube is held with your hand, your hand is in harm's way if the needle slips off the tube top when puncturing it with the syringe. Do not force the blood into the tube. This technique maintains the proper ratio of blood to anticoagulant.

Do not remove the rubber stoppers. Running blood down the side of the tube after removing the stopper is not recommended because aerosols and splattering of blood can occur.

Evacuated Tube Sample Collection

The evacuated tube system is an improvement over the syringe method, yet maintains many similarities. When using the syringe method, as the syringe plunger is pulled, a vacuum is created. With

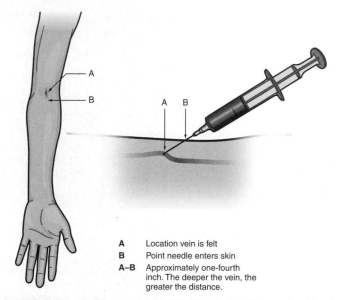

A	Location vein is felt
B	Point needle enters skin
A–B	Approximately one-fourth inch. The deeper the vein, the greater the distance.

FIGURE 2.10 *Position at which to enter the skin. Left diagram, location at which vein is felt (A); point at which needle enters the skin (B). Right diagram, distance between A and B is approximately ¼ inch. The deeper the vein, the greater the distance.*
© Cengage Learning 2013

the evacuated tube system, the vacuum is already in the tube. Another advantage of the evacuated tube system is that with multiple blood samples, syringes do not need to be changed; only the tubes need to be changed. This creates the advantage of a closed system; there is no transferring of blood from the syringe to a tube.

The similarity between the evacuated tube system and the syringe system is that the holder and needle are held in the same manner. A syringe is held in a manner to allow the phlebotomist access to pull on the plunger. In the evacuated system, access must be allowed for one tube to be pulled out and another inserted. The hand that pulls on the plunger of the syringe is the hand that changes tubes with the evacuated system.

PROCEDURE 2.3 Venipuncture by Syringe

Principle:

To obtain venous blood acceptable for laboratory testing as required by a physician. Venous blood collected is to be aliquoted into evacuated tubes and/or special collection containers.

Materials:

Disposable gloves

Goggles and mask

Syringe, varies in size

Disposable needle for syringe, 21 or 22 gauge

Evacuated tube(s) or special collection tube(s)

Tourniquet

70 percent isopropyl alcohol swab

Gauze or cotton balls

Adhesive bandage or tape

Sharps container

Transfer device

Procedure:

1. Identify the patient. *Inpatient:* Ask the patient his or her name, to spell his or her last name, and verify the identification bracelet name and hospital number with the computer label or requisition information. *Outpatient:* Ask the patient his or her name, to spell his or her last name, and verify these with the computer label or requisition information.

continues

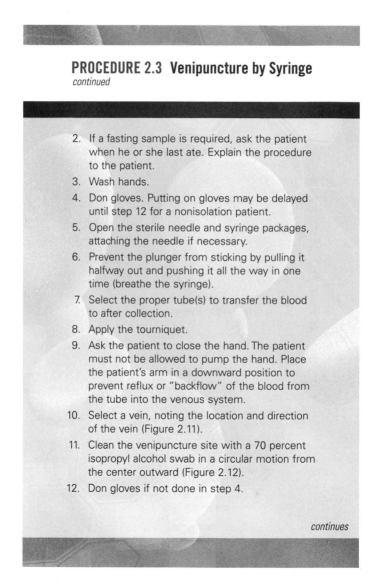

PROCEDURE 2.3 Venipuncture by Syringe
continued

2. If a fasting sample is required, ask the patient when he or she last ate. Explain the procedure to the patient.

3. Wash hands.

4. Don gloves. Putting on gloves may be delayed until step 12 for a nonisolation patient.

5. Open the sterile needle and syringe packages, attaching the needle if necessary.

6. Prevent the plunger from sticking by pulling it halfway out and pushing it all the way in one time (breathe the syringe).

7. Select the proper tube(s) to transfer the blood to after collection.

8. Apply the tourniquet.

9. Ask the patient to close the hand. The patient must not be allowed to pump the hand. Place the patient's arm in a downward position to prevent reflux or "backflow" of the blood from the tube into the venous system.

10. Select a vein, noting the location and direction of the vein (Figure 2.11).

11. Clean the venipuncture site with a 70 percent isopropyl alcohol swab in a circular motion from the center outward (Figure 2.12).

12. Don gloves if not done in step 4.

continues

PROCEDURE 2.3 Venipuncture by Syringe
continued

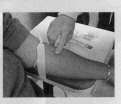

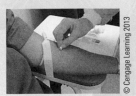

FIGURE 2.11 *Feel for a vein.*

FIGURE 2.12 *Clean the site with isopropyl alcohol.*

© Cengage Learning 2013

13. Do not touch the venipuncture site. If there is a potential for blood spatter, goggles and a mask must be worn.

14. Draw the skin taut with your thumb. Place the thumb 1 to 2 inches below the puncture site (Figure 2.13).

15. With the bevel up, line up the needle with the vein and perform the venipuncture (Figure 2.14).

16. Do not enter the vein at the exact location where the vein is felt. Enter the vein approximately 0.5 cm (¼ inch) below the vein location. The location where the vein was palpated is the point where the bevel of the needle must be in the vein (see Figure 2.10). Push the needle into the skin. A sensation of resistance will be followed by easy penetration as the vein is entered. This is known as feeling the "pop." Once this point is reached, stop and do not move.

continues

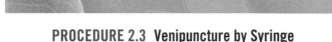

PROCEDURE 2.3 Venipuncture by Syringe
continued

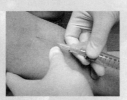 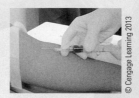

© Cengage Learning 2013

FIGURE 2.13 *Draw the skin taut with your thumb.*

FIGURE 2.14 *Perform the venipuncture. Secure the syringe with one hand and pull on the plunger with the other hand.*

17. Using the opposite hand, pull on the plunger of the syringe. Pull gently and only as fast as the syringe will fill with blood. Pulling too hard or fast will cause temporary collapse of the vein. If the vein does collapse, stop pulling on the plunger and let the vein refill with blood.

18. Pull the plunger back until the desired amount of blood has been obtained.

19. Ask the patient to open the hand.

20. Release the tourniquet.

21. Lightly place a gauze square or cotton ball above the venipuncture site.

22. Remove the needle from the arm.

23. Activate the safety shield over the needle.

continues

PROCEDURE 2.3 Venipuncture by Syringe
continued

24. Apply pressure to the site for 3 to 5 minutes.
    The patient may assist if able by elevating the
    arm above the heart level. The patient should
    not bend his or her arm.

25. Aliquot blood into the appropriate tubes. Re-
    move the needle from the syringe, and then
    discard the needle into the sharps container.
    Attach the transfer device. Fill the tubes via
    the transfer device following the correct order
    of draw (Figure 2.15). Allow blood to enter the

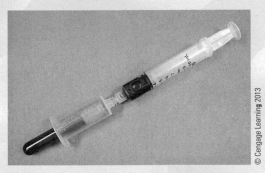

© Cengage Learning 2013

FIGURE 2.15   *Use of a transfer device to fill evacuated tubes.*

continues

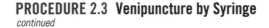

PROCEDURE 2.3 Venipuncture by Syringe
continued

tube until flow stops. Mix if any anticoagulant or additive is present. Gently inverting the tube five to eight times provides adequate mixing without causing hemolysis. Alternately, place the appropriate tube(s) in a test tube rack. Puncture the stopper of the evacuated tube with the syringe needle and allow blood to enter the tube until flow stops (Figure 2.16). Invert the tube(s) if any anticoagulant is present.

26. Dispose of the syringe and transfer device into the sharps container. Do not disconnect the syringe from the transfer device or needle before disposal. Dispose of the devices intact.

27. Discard the gauze and other waste in the biohazard containers.

28. Label all tubes before leaving the patient.

29. Check the puncture site. Apply adhesive bandage. If the patient is an infant, the use of the bandage should be eliminated.

30. Remove gloves and wash hands.

31. Thank the patient and transport the sample(s) to the laboratory.

continues

PROCEDURE 2.3 Venipuncture by Syringe
continued

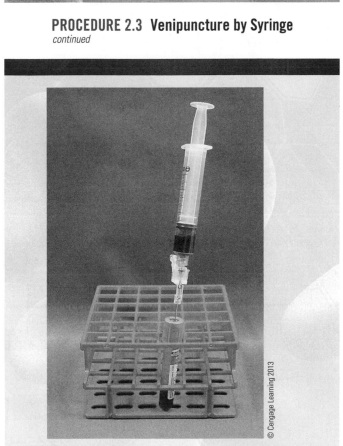

© Cengage Learning 2013

FIGURE 2.16 *Puncture the stopper of the evacuated tube with the syringe needle and allow blood to enter the tube until flow stops.*

The procedure for venipuncture with the evacuated tube system follows the same steps as those for the syringe method with only slight variation (Procedure 2.4).

Butterfly Collection System

The butterfly system maintains many similarities to the evacuated system. The butterfly provides the convenience of evacuated tubes but offers the flexibility to use a syringe if needed. What most phlebotomists like about the butterfly system is that when the needle enters the vein there is a "flash" of blood where the tubing is attached to the needle. This flash gives the phlebotomist a visual that the vein has been accessed. For an experienced phlebotomist, this visual flash is not necessary for most patients and a regular needle can be used.

Using the butterfly system with each patient is more costly than the regular needle system. Therefore, the butterfly system should be limited to patients who have small veins such as pediatric patients or oncology patients.

One concern with the butterfly collection system is the air in the tubing after the venipuncture has been performed. The first tube pulls the air from the tubing, resulting in a tube that is approximately 0.5 milliliter short of the correct amount of blood. This is not a problem for most tests. However, a light blue–stoppered tube must maintain the 1:9 ratio of anticoagulant to blood for accurate testing from that tube. When the first tube to be collected is a light blue–stoppered tube, a discard tube (a red-stoppered tube with no additive or another light blue–stoppered tube) must be collected to pull the air from the tubing. A discard tube that has any additive cannot be used because of the carryover of the additive into the light blue–stoppered tube.

The procedures for venipuncture with the butterfly system follows the same steps as those for the evacuated tube system with only slight variation (Procedures 2.5 and 2.6).

The Unsuccessful Venipuncture

When a blood sample cannot be obtained, it may be necessary to change the position of the needle. Rotate the needle half a turn. The bevel of the needle may be against the wall of the vein. If the needle

PROCEDURE 2.4 Venipuncture by Evacuated Tube System

Principle:
To obtain venous blood acceptable for laboratory testing as required by a physician. Venous blood is collected by evacuated tubes. The volume of blood is dependent on the size of the tube and on test requirements.

Materials:
Gloves

Goggles and mask

Evacuated tube holder

Disposable needle for evacuated system, 20, 21, or 22 gauge

Evacuated tube(s) or special collection tube(s)

Tourniquet

70 percent isopropyl alcohol swab

Gauze or cotton balls

Adhesive bandage or tape

Sharps container

Procedure:

1. Identify the patient. *Inpatient:* Ask the patient his or her name, to spell his or her last name, and verify the identification bracelet name and hospital number with the computer label or requisition information. *Outpatient:* Ask the

continues

PROCEDURE 2.4 Venipuncture by Evacuated Tube System *continued*

patient his or her name, to spell his or her last name, and verify these with the computer label or requisition information.

2. If a fasting sample is required, ask the patient when he or she last ate.

3. Wash hands.

4. Don gloves. Putting on gloves may be delayed until step 12 for nonisolation patients.

5. Collect the equipment.

6. Break the needle seal. Thread the appropriate needle into the holder, using the needle sheath as a wrench.

7. Before using, tap all tubes that contain additives to ensure that all the additive is dislodged from the stopper and wall of the tube.

8. Insert the tube into the holder until the needle slightly enters the stopper. Avoid pushing the needle beyond the recessed guideline because a loss of vacuum may result. If the tube retracts slightly, leave it in the retracted position to avoid prematurely puncturing the rubber stopper.

9. Apply the tourniquet.

10. Ask the patient to close the hand. The patient must not be allowed to pump the hand. Place the patient's arm in a downward position to

continues

PROCEDURE 2.4 Venipuncture by Evacuated Tube System *continued*

prevent reflux or "backflow" of the blood from the tube into the venous system.

11. Feel for a vein, noting its location and direction (Figure 2.17).

12. Clean the venipuncture site with a 70 percent isopropyl alcohol swab in a circular motion from the center outward.

13. Don gloves if not done in step 4.

14. Do not touch the venipuncture site. If there is a potential for blood spatter, goggles and a mask must be worn.

15. Draw the skin taut with your thumb. Place the thumb 1 to 2 inches below the puncture site.

16. With the bevel up, line up the needle with the vein while holding the skin taut with your thumb. Perform the venipuncture (Figure 2.18). Remove your hand from drawing the skin taut (Figure 2.19). Grasp the flange of the evacuated tube holder, and push the tube forward until the needle punctures the stopper (Figure 2.20). You should not change hands while performing the venipuncture. The hand you perform the venipuncture with is the hand that holds the evacuated tube holder. This provides stability for the phlebotomist and the comfort of human touch to the patient. The opposite hand manipulates the tubes.

continues

PROCEDURE 2.4 Venipuncture by Evacuated Tube System *continued*

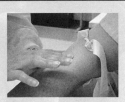

FIGURE 2.17   *Feel for vein direction and location.*

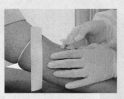

FIGURE 2.18   *Insert the needle while holding the skin taut with your thumb.*

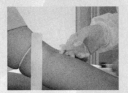

FIGURE 2.19   *Remove your hand from holding the skin taut.*

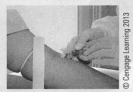

FIGURE 2.20   *Insert the tubes into the holder in the correct order of draw.*

© Cengage Learning 2013

17. Do not enter the vein at the exact location where the vein is felt. Enter the vein approximately 0.5 cm (¼ inch) below the vein location. The location that the vein was palpated is the point where the bevel of the needle must be in the vein. Push the needle into the skin.

continues

PROCEDURE 2.4 **Venipuncture by Evacuated Tube System** *continued*

A sensation of resistance will be followed by easy penetration as the vein is entered. This is known as feeling the "pop." Once this point is reached, stop and do not move.

18. Fill the tube until the vacuum is exhausted and blood flow into the tube ceases (Figure 2.21). This ensures the proper blood-to-anticoagulant ratio. Remove the tube from the holder. While securely grasping the evacuated tube holder with one hand, use the flange on the tube holder to give leverage to change the tubes. The shutoff valve re-covers the point, stopping the flow of blood until the next tube of blood is inserted. Fill the remaining tubes following the correct order of draw.

19. Immediately after filling, invert each tube that contains an additive. Gently inverting the tube five to eight times provides adequate mixing

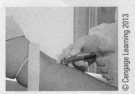

© Cengage Learning 2013

FIGURE 2.21 *Fill tube until vacuum is exhausted.*

continues

PROCEDURE 2.4 Venipuncture by Evacuated Tube System *continued*

without causing hemolysis. Do not shake the tube.

20. Ask the patient to open the hand.

21. Release the tourniquet.

22. Lightly place a gauze square or cotton ball above the venipuncture site.

23. Remove the needle from the arm. Be certain that the last tube drawn has been removed from the holder before removing the needle. This prevents blood droplets from falling off the tip of the needle.

24. Activate the safety shield on the needle.

25. Dispose of the needle and holder in a sharps container.

26. Apply pressure to the site for 3 to 5 minutes. The patient may assist if able and elevate the arm above the heart to reduce blood flow.

27. Label all tubes at the patient's side before leaving the patient.

28. Check the puncture site. Apply adhesive bandage. If the patient is an infant, the use of the bandage should be eliminated.

29. Remove gloves and wash hands.

30. Thank the patient and transport the sample(s) to the laboratory.

PROCEDURE 2.5 Antecubital Vein Venipuncture by Butterfly (Winged Infusion Set) Collection System Using Evacuated Tubes

Principle:

To obtain venous blood acceptable for laboratory testing as required by a physician. The amount of the venous blood sample is dependent on the size of the tube and the test requirements.

Materials:

Gloves

Goggles and mask

Evacuated tube holder

Butterfly needle system, 21- or 23-gauge needle with or without Luer adapter

Syringe if not using Luer adapter on butterfly needle

Evacuated tube(s) or special collection tube(s)

Tourniquet

70 percent isopropyl alcohol swab

Gauze or cotton balls

Adhesive bandage or tape

Sharps container

Procedure:

1. Identify the patient. *Inpatient:* Ask the patient his or her name, to spell his or her last name, and verify the identification bracelet name and hospital number with the computer label or

continues

PROCEDURE 2.5 Antecubital Vein Venipuncture by Butterfly (Winged Infusion Set) Collection System Using Evacuated Tubes
continued

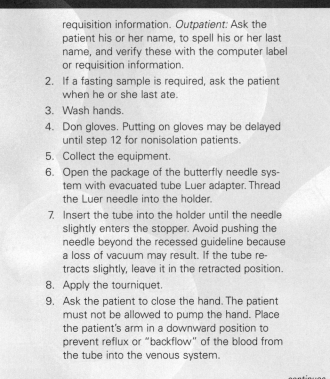

requisition information. *Outpatient:* Ask the patient his or her name, to spell his or her last name, and verify these with the computer label or requisition information.

2. If a fasting sample is required, ask the patient when he or she last ate.

3. Wash hands.

4. Don gloves. Putting on gloves may be delayed until step 12 for nonisolation patients.

5. Collect the equipment.

6. Open the package of the butterfly needle system with evacuated tube Luer adapter. Thread the Luer needle into the holder.

7. Insert the tube into the holder until the needle slightly enters the stopper. Avoid pushing the needle beyond the recessed guideline because a loss of vacuum may result. If the tube retracts slightly, leave it in the retracted position.

8. Apply the tourniquet.

9. Ask the patient to close the hand. The patient must not be allowed to pump the hand. Place the patient's arm in a downward position to prevent reflux or "backflow" of the blood from the tube into the venous system.

continues

PROCEDURE 2.5 Antecubital Vein Venipuncture by Butterfly (Winged Infusion Set) Collection System Using Evacuated Tubes

continued

10. Feel for a vein, noting its location and direction (Figure 2.22).

11. Clean the venipuncture site with a 70 percent isopropyl alcohol swab in a circular motion from the center outward (Figure 2.23).

12. Don gloves if not done in step 4.

13. Do not touch the venipuncture site. If there is a potential for blood spatter, goggles and a mask must be worn.

14. Draw the skin taut with your thumb. Place your thumb 1 to 2 inches below the puncture site.

15. Hold the butterfly with the bevel up. Line up the needle with the vein and perform the venipuncture (Figure 2.24).

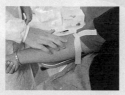

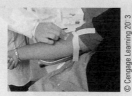

© Cengage Learning 20·3

FIGURE 2.22 *Feel for a vein.*

FIGURE 2.23 *Clean the venipuncture site with isopropyl alcohol.*

continues

PROCEDURE 2.5 Antecubital Vein Venipuncture by Butterfly (Winged Infusion Set) Collection System Using Evacuated Tubes
continued

16. Do not enter the vein at the exact location where the vein is felt. Enter the vein approximately 0.5 cm (¼ inch) below the vein location. The location where the vein was palpated is the point where the bevel of the needle must be in the vein. Push the needle into the skin. A sensation of resistance will be followed by easy penetration as the vein is entered. This is known as feeling the "pop." Once this point is reached, you should see a flash of blood in the needle tubing (Figure 2.25). Stop and do not move.

17. Remove your hand from drawing the skin taut. Grasp the flange of the evacuated tube holder and push the tube forward until the butt end of

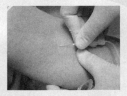

FIGURE 2.24 *Perform the venipuncture.*

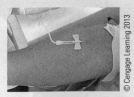

FIGURE 2.25 *When the needle enters the vein, you should see a "flash" of blood.*

© Cengage Learning 2013

continues

PROCEDURE 2.5 Antecubital Vein Venipuncture by Butterfly (Winged Infusion Set) Collection System Using Evacuated Tubes
continued

the needle punctures the stopper (Figure 2.26). Do not change hands while performing the venipuncture. The hand performing the venipuncture is the hand that holds the butterfly needle. The opposite hand manipulates the tubes.

18. Fill the tube until the vacuum is exhausted and blood flow into the tube ceases. This ensures the proper blood-to-anticoagulant ratio. Due to air in the tubing, a loss of approximately 0.5 milliliter of blood will result when collecting the initial evacuated tube.

19. When the blood flow ceases, remove the tube from the holder. While securely grasping the evacuated tube holder with one hand, use the flange on the tube holder to give leverage to

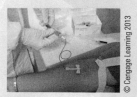

© Cengage Learning 2013

FIGURE 2.26 *Insert the evacuated tube into the holder.*

continues

PROCEDURE 2.5 Antecubital Vein Venipuncture by Butterfly (Winged Infusion Set) Collection System Using Evacuated Tubes

continued

change the tubes. Insert the next tube into the holder according to the correct order of draw. The shutoff valve re-covers the point, stopping the flow of blood until the next tube of blood is inserted.

20. Immediately after drawing, invert each tube that contains an additive. Gently inverting the tube five to eight times provides adequate mixing without causing hemolysis. Do not shake the tubes.

21. Ask the patient to open the hand.

22. Release the tourniquet (Figure 2.27).

23. Remove the last tube to draw from the holder (Figure 2.28).

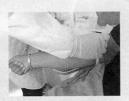

FIGURE 2.27 *Release the tourniquet.*

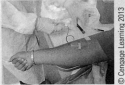

© Cengage Learning 2013

FIGURE 2.28 *Remove the last tube from the holder.*

continues

PROCEDURE 2.5 Antecubital Vein Venipuncture by Butterfly (Winged Infusion Set) Collection System Using Evacuated Tubes
continued

24. Lightly place a gauze square or cotton ball above the venipuncture site.

25. Remove the needle from the arm. Be certain that the last tube drawn has been removed from the holder before removing the needle (Figure 2.29). This prevents blood from dripping out of the tip of the needle. Note: Some butterfly needles have a push-button retraction of the needle. With these devices, the push button is pressed and the needle retracts from the patient, therefore activating the safety feature.

26. Activate the safety shield on the needle if not activated by push button (Figure 2.30).

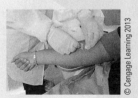

© Cengage Learning 2013

FIGURE 2.29 *Remove the butterfly needle from the arm.*

continues

PROCEDURE 2.5 Antecubital Vein Venipuncture by Butterfly (Winged Infusion Set) Collection System Using Evacuated Tubes
continued

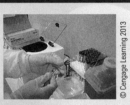

FIGURE 2.30 *Activate the safety shield if not previously activated with a push-button device.*

27. Apply pressure to the site for 3 to 5 minutes. The patient may assist if able. The arm should be elevated to reduce blood flow.

28. Dispose of the needle and holder in a sharps container. When disposing, insert the needle end of the device first and allow the tubing and holder to drop into the container.

29. Label all the tubes at the patient's side before leaving the room.

30. Check the puncture site. Apply adhesive bandage. If the patient is an infant, the use of the bandage should be eliminated.

31. Remove gloves and wash hands.

32. Thank the patient and transport the sample(s) to the laboratory.

PROCEDURE 2.6 Hand Vein Venipuncture by Butterfly (Winged Infusion Set) Collection System Using a Syringe

Principle:

To obtain venous blood acceptable for laboratory testing as required by a physician.

Sample:

Venous blood collected by evacuated tubes. Volume of blood dependent on size of tube and test requirements.

Materials:

Evacuated tube holder

Disposable butterfly needle with safety shield, 21 or 23 gauge

10-mL to 15-mL syringe

Transfer device

Tourniquot

70 percent isopropyl alcohol swab

Gauze or cotton balls

Adhesive bandage or tape

Disposable gloves

Biohazard sharps container

Safety glasses and mask

Procedure:

1. Identify the patient. *Inpatient:* Ask the patient his or her name, to spell his or her last name, and verify the identification bracelet name and

continues

PROCEDURE 2.6 Hand Vein Venipuncture by Butterfly (Winged Infusion Set) Collection System Using a Syringe *continued*

    hospital number with the computer label or requisition information. *Outpatient:* Ask the patient his or her name, to spell his or her last name, and verify these with the computer label or requisition information.

2. If a fasting sample is required, ask the patient when he or she last ate. Explain the procedure to the patient.

3. Collect the equipment. Wash hands. Put on gloves.

4. Open the package containing the butterfly needle system. Connect the syringe to the butterfly needle system (Figure 2.31).

5. Apply the tourniquet.

6. Ask the patient to close the hand. The patient must not be allowed to pump the hand. Place

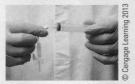

© Cengage Learning 2013

FIGURE 2.31 *Connect the syringe to the butterfly needle system.*

continues

PROCEDURE 2.6 Hand Vein Venipuncture by Butterfly (Winged Infusion Set) Collection System Using a Syringe *continued*

the patient's arm in a downward position to prevent reflux or "backflow" of the blood from the tube into the venous system (Figure 2.32).

7. Feel for a vein, noting its location and direction.

8. Clean the venipuncture with a 70 percent isopropyl alcohol swab (Figure 2.33).

9. Put on gloves while the alcohol is drying if you did not do so in step 3. Do not touch the venipuncture site.

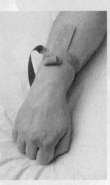

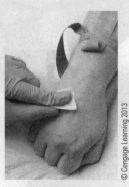

© Cengage Learning 2013

FIGURE 2.32 *Apply the tourniquet. Ask the patient to close his or her hand.*

FIGURE 2.33 *Clean the venipuncture site.*

continues

PROCEDURE 2.6 Hand Vein Venipuncture by Butterfly (Winged Infusion Set) Collection System Using a Syringe *continued*

10. Draw the patient's skin taut with your thumb. The thumb should be slightly below the puncture site and a little to the side for maximum access to the vein.

11. With the bevel up, line up the needle with the vein while holding the skin taut. Perform the venipuncture at a 5- to 10-degree angle (Figure 2.34). When the needle enters the vein, you should see a "flash" of blood.

12. Continue holding the needle in position. Gently pull on the syringe with the other hand, allowing the syringe to fill (Figure 2.35).

13. When the syringe is filled to the desired amount, have the patient open the hand and release the tourniquet. Place a cotton ball or gauze above the venipuncture site and remove the needle (Figure 2.36). Note: Some butterfly needles have a push-button retraction of the needle. With these devices, the push button is pressed and the needle retracts from the patient, therefore activating the safety feature.

14. Activate the safety shield over the needle if not activated by push-button (Figure 2.37).

continues

PROCEDURE 2.6 Hand Vein Venipuncture by Butterfly (Winged Infusion Set) Collection System Using a Syringe *continued*

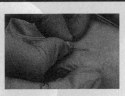

FIGURE 2.34 *Perform the venipuncture at a 5- to 10-degree angle.*

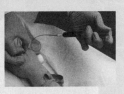

FIGURE 2.35 *Gently pull on the syringe with the other hand, allowing the syringe to fill.*

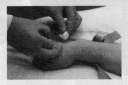

FIGURE 2.36 *When the syringe is filled to the desired amount, have the patient open his or her hand and release the tourniquet. Place a cotton ball or gauze above the venipuncture site and remove the needle.*

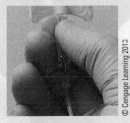

© Cengage Learning 2013

FIGURE 2.37 *Activate the safety shield if not previously activated with a push-button device.*

continues

PROCEDURE 2.6 Hand Vein Venipuncture by Butterfly (Winged Infusion Set) Collection System Using a Syringe *continued*

15. Apply pressure to the site, and ask the patient if he or she can continue to hold pressure (Figure 2.38).

16. Disconnect the syringe from the butterfly device.

17. Dispose of the butterfly device in the sharps container (Figure 2.39).

18. Fill the evacuated tubes in the correct order of draw from the syringe using a transfer device. Fill each tube until the vacuum is

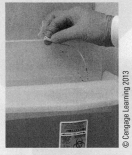

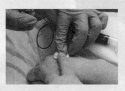

© Cengage Learning 2013

FIGURE 2.38 *Apply pressure to the site, and ask the patient if he or she can continue to hold pressure.*

FIGURE 2.39 *Dispose of the butterfly device in the sharps container.*

continues

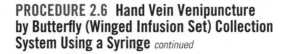

PROCEDURE 2.6 Hand Vein Venipuncture by Butterfly (Winged Infusion Set) Collection System Using a Syringe *continued*

    exhausted and blood flow into the tube ceases, ensuring the proper blood-to-anticoagulant ratio.

19. Mix each tube that contains an additive immediately after filling. Gently inverting the tube five to eight times provides adequate mixing without causing hemolysis.

20. Recheck the identification bracelet with the labels or requisitions.

21. Label all tubes.

22. Check the puncture site. Apply adhesive bandage. If the patient is an infant, the use of the bandage should be eliminated.

23. Remove gloves and wash hands.

24. Thank the patient and transport the sample(s) to the laboratory.

has not penetrated the vein far enough, advance it farther into the vein. Only advance slightly; a small change may be the difference between a failed and a successful venipuncture. If the needle has penetrated too far into the vein, pull back a little. Always "bail out" slowly when the venipuncture has been unsuccessful. The blood often may start coming just as it seems the needle is ready to come out of the skin. The tube used may not have sufficient vacuum. Try another tube before withdrawing the needle.

The tourniquet could have been on too tight, stopping the flow of blood. Reapply the tourniquet loosely. An alternative to a tourniquet is a blood pressure cuff inflated to between the patient's systolic and diastolic pressure. The cuff provides a larger surface area to apply pressure, and the pressure can be regulated. This often brings veins to the surface when other methods have failed.

Probing of the site is not recommended. Probing is painful to the patient and may cause a hematoma. Never attempt a venipuncture more than two times. If a blood sample cannot be obtained after two attempts, perform a microcollection if possible. Otherwise have another person attempt the draw. Notify the patient's physician if two attempts have been unsuccessful and a microcollection is not possible.

Criteria for Re-collection or Rejection of a Sample

The primary goal of the phlebotomist collecting the blood sample is to provide an acceptable sample for laboratory testing as required by the physician. There are certain general criteria that must be met for a sample to be acceptable. If the criteria are not met, the sample is rejected and another venipuncture of the patient must be performed.

This list is not inclusive. The type of sample that is acceptable and the volume required is determined by the procedure ordered. Another sample is often done to recheck results on a patient. The quality control checks done by the laboratory may indicate that the results are valid. If the results do not agree with what the physician feels is the patient's diagnosis, the blood sample may need to be redrawn to confirm the results. This is accomplished by either retesting the sample or collecting another sample. This will either reconfirm that the correct sample was drawn or indicate that the patient's test results changed significantly.

QUALITY ASSURANCE FOR SAMPLES

1. Each sample must have its own label attached to the sample's primary container.
2. Labels must have the patient's complete name and identification number.
3. Samples in syringes with needles still attached are unacceptable.
4. All samples must be in their appropriate anticoagulant.
5. Anticoagulated blood collection tubes must be at least 75 percent full. All coagulation blood collection tubes (light-blue stoppers, such as for prothrombin time [PT] and partial thromboplastin time [PTT]) must be 100 percent full.
6. Anticoagulated blood samples must be free of clots.
7. Certain tests require samples to be free of hemolysis and lipemia.
8. The sample may need to be recollected if the results do not agree with what the physician feels is the diagnosis of the patient.

Factors Affecting Laboratory Values

Numerous variables can affect test results. The samples are tested by analytical instruments that give accurate and precise results. These results only accurately reflect what is wrong with the patient if the sample is correctly collected. A correctly collected sample is the responsibility of the phlebotomist. Patient physiological factors may also contribute to inaccurate results.

The patient can knowingly or unknowingly alter the results by certain actions. An example of this occurs when patients say they have had nothing to eat or drink, but they have had a cup of coffee. The patient is often under the misconception that black coffee without sugar is not a problem. Coffee and smoking affect the metabolism and therefore can alter test results.

FACTORS THAT CAN ALTER RESULTS

Patient-controlled factors that can alter test results include the following:

1. Fasting—If the patient is not in a fasting state when he or she should have been, results of tests will not be accurate. Glucose values will be elevated.

2. Prolonged fasting—Fasting for more than 14 hours causes increases and decreases in certain tests.

   Increases: amino acids, bilirubin, fatty acids, glucagon, growth hormone, ketones, lactate, triglycerides

   Decreases: glucose, high-density lipoprotein (HDL) cholesterol, insulin, lactate dehydrogenase (LDH), T3

3. Stress—Stress can have an effect. In children, violent crying before a sample is collected raises the white blood cell (WBC) count up to 146 percent.

4. Exercise—Strenuous short-term exercise can make the heart work harder and increase the heart enzymes and WBC count.

Phlebotomist-controlled factors include the following:

1. Tourniquet—Hemoconcentration, a change in chemical concentration, which can result from a tourniquet tied too tightly, or the tourniquet being left on longer than 1 minute. This causes elevated levels of potassium, total protein, calcium, bilirubin, alanine aminotransferase (ALT), aspartate aminotransferase (AST), cholesterol, triglycerides, albumin, hemoglobin, and cell counts.

2. Heparin—Using an incorrect heparin tube can interfere with tests being run.

3. Correct volume—Not enough blood drawn causes an improper anticoagulant-to-blood ratio that can change the size of the cells and therefore cause a variation in test results.

4. Inappropriate use of gel tubes—The gel can affect results of some therapeutic drug levels and blood bank testing.

5. Test exposed to light—Some tests must not be exposed to light. Vitamin E and bilirubin will have lower values after 1 hour of exposure to light. Amber tubes or foil-wrapped tubes will protect the sample.

6. Incomplete sterilization of blood culture collection site—The incomplete sterilization of blood culture collection sites will result in a false positive blood culture. This causes a prolonged patient stay and increased cost to the patient.

7. Diurnal rhythm—Some samples must be drawn at timed intervals because of medication or diurnal rhythm. The exact time of collection must also be noted on the sample.

Chilling or Warming of Samples

Certain samples must be chilled or kept warmed immediately after collection. To chill a sample, place the blood tube into an ice and water mixture as it is withdrawn from the evacuated tube holder (Figure 2.40). The mixture of ice and water provides an increased surface area to cool the sample. This sample should then be placed in a biohazard bag for transport. Make sure that the label will not come

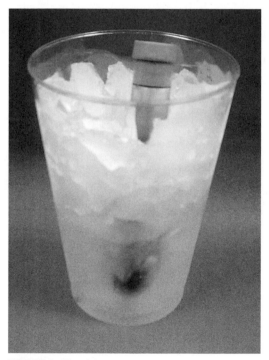

FIGURE 2.40 *Icing a sample in ice and water solution.*
© Cengage Learning 2013

off in the water and the ink will not run, leaving the label unreadable. If this is the case, label the tube, place the tube in a bag, and then place this tube in the ice and water mixture.

To keep a sample warm, wrap an infant heel warmer around the sample (Figure 2.41). Any delay in icing or warming the sample will alter test results. The longer the delay, the greater the change. The phlebotomist must refer to the laboratory directory of service to determine if a sample needs to be iced or warmed.

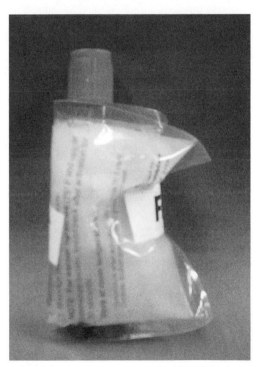

FIGURE 2.41   *Warming a sample with an infant heel warmer.*
© Cengage Learning 2013

Blood Cultures

Blood cultures are collected whenever it is suspected that a patient has septicemia (Procedure 2.7). Septicemia is a condition in which microorganisms (mainly bacteria) circulate and multiply in the patient's blood. Because blood is normally sterile, the presence of microorganisms and their products is very serious and can result in death. The blood is collected and placed in a bottle that contains a solution that enhances the growth of significant microorganisms. An anticoagulant is also present. The microorganisms can then be cultured and identified so the most effective antibiotic treatment can be started.

If blood cultures are to be collected after antimicrobial treatment has started, the blood culture must be drawn in a special bottle containing a solution to inactivate the antimicrobial agent. This will then allow the bacteria to grow.

The volume of blood needed is critical to optimum recovery of the microorganisms. From 8 to 10 milliliters of blood is to be placed in the bottle. The optimum amount of blood varies depending on the manufacturer of the blood culture bottles. Adult draws usually need a total of 20 milliliters for the best recovery of microorganisms. Any lesser amount will reduce the recovery rate and lengthen the time to recovery. For infants and children, 1 to 4 milliliters of blood in a pediatric bottle is sufficient.

For adults, blood cultures are drawn in sets of two bottles. One bottle is the aerobic bottle for those microorganisms that need oxygen to grow. The second bottle is an anaerobic bottle for the microorganisms requiring an environment without oxygen. A set of blood cultures traditionally is collected at the height of the patient's fever. This is when the microorganisms were thought to be at their greatest number in the blood. With the new high-recovery blood culture bottles being used, drawing of the blood at the height of the fever is not as critical. Even during a low point of the fever, the microorganisms are present in sufficient number for rapid growth. Two blood culture sets are usually sufficient for recovery of significant microorganisms. These two sets consist of an aerobic and anaerobic blood culture collected from one patient site, such as the left arm, and another set of aerobic and anaerobic bottles collected from an alternate location. Ideally, the two sets are collected before starting antibiotic therapy.

The most critical step in collecting a blood culture is the proper cleaning of the site when doing a venipuncture. The site must be as clean as possible to avoid contaminating the blood culture with skin surface microorganisms and producing a false-positive blood culture. Commercial kits are available that can help with the cleaning (Figure 2.42).

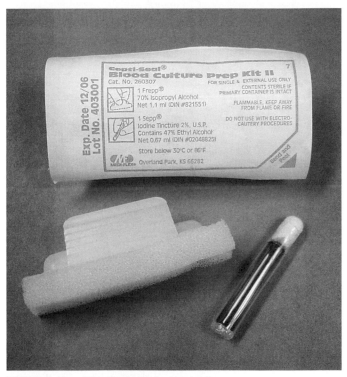

FIGURE 2.42 *Skin cleaning kit for blood cultures.*
© Cengage Learning 2013

PROCEDURE 2.7 Blood Culture Collection with a Butterfly (Winged Infusion Set)

Principle:
To obtain venous blood acceptable for laboratory testing as required by a physician. Venous blood is collected by a butterfly needle system directly into blood culture containers.

Materials:
Gloves

Goggles and mask

Evacuated tube holder

Butterfly needle system, 21- or 23-gauge needle with or without Luer adapter

Syringe if not using Luer adapter on butterfly needle

22-gauge syringe needle

Tube holder for blood culture bottles

Aerobic and anaerobic blood culture bottles

Blood culture skin cleaning kit

Tourniquet

70 percent isopropyl alcohol swab

Gauze or cotton balls

Adhesive bandage or tape

Sharps container

Procedure:

1. Identify the patient. *Inpatient:* Ask the patient his or her name, to spell his or her last name,

continues

PROCEDURE 2.7 Blood Culture Collection with a Butterfly (Winged Infusion Set) *continued*

    and verify the identification bracelet name and hospital number with the computer label or requisition information. *Outpatient:* Ask the patient his or her name, to spell his or her last name, and verify these with the computer label or requisition information.

2. Wash hands and collect the equipment.

3. Don gloves. Putting on gloves may be delayed until step 12 for nonisolation patients.

4. Open the package of the butterfly needle system with evacuated tube Luer adapter.

5. Thread the Luer needle into the special blood culture bottle holder (Figure 2.43).

6. The recommended fill for each blood culture bottle is 8 to 10 milliliters of blood. Mark each bottle 8 to 10 milliliters above the level of the culture media, using the scale on the side of the bottle.

7. Remove the plastic flip top or overcap from the aerobic and anaerobic bottles and disinfect the top of the bottles with an alcohol pad.

8. Apply the tourniquet.

9. Ask the patient to close the hand. The patient must not be allowed to pump the hand. If possible, place the patient's arm in a downward position.

continues

PROCEDURE 2.7 Blood Culture Collection with a Butterfly (Winged Infusion Set) *continued*

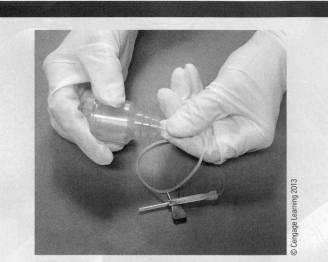

© Cengage Learning 2013

FIGURE 2.43 *Attaching the butterfly to the special blood culture bottle holder.*

10. Feel for a vein, noting its location and direction.
11. Verify that the patient is not allergic to iodine. Clean the venipuncture site using the special blood culture cleaning kit. Scrub with an alcohol scrub pad; allow the alcohol to dry, then clean with an iodine solution in a circular motion from

continues

PROCEDURE 2.7 Blood Culture Collection with a Butterfly (Winged Infusion Set) *continued*

        the center outward. Allow sufficient time for the iodine to dry. Depending on the type of iodine used this can be 30 to 60 seconds. The drying action helps kill the skin surface bacteria.

12. Don gloves if not done in step 3.

13. Do not touch the venipuncture site. If there is a potential for blood spatter, goggles and a mask must be worn.

14. Draw the skin taut with your thumb. Place your thumb 1 to 2 inches below the puncture site.

15. Hold the butterfly with the bevel up. With the bevel up, line up the needle with the vein and perform the venipuncture.

16. Do not enter the vein at the exact location where the vein is felt. Enter the vein approximately 0.5 cm (¼ inch) below the vein location. The location where the vein was palpated is the point where the bevel of the needle must be in the vein. Push the needle into the skin. A sensation of resistance will be followed by easy penetration as the vein is entered. This is known as feeling the "pop." Once this point is reached, you should see a flash of blood in the needle tubing. Stop and do not move.

17. Remove your hand from drawing the skin taut. Grasp the tube holder and place it over the top

continues

PROCEDURE 2.7 Blood Culture Collection with a Butterfly (Winged Infusion Set) *continued*

of the aerobic blood culture bottle (Figure 2.44). Push the holder down to allow blood to enter the bottle. Remove the holder when the bottle volume reaches the previously marked line.

18. Fill the anaerobic bottle second. Due to air in the tubing, the aerobic bottle must be filled first to avoid contaminating the anaerobic bottle.

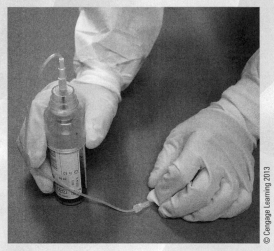

FIGURE 2.44   *Proper placement of the holder on the blood culture bottle.*

© Cengage Learning 2013

continues

PROCEDURE 2.7 Blood Culture Collection with a Butterfly (Winged Infusion Set) *continued*

19. Ask the patient to open the hand.

20. Release the tourniquet.

21. Lightly place a gauze square or cotton ball above the venipuncture site.

22. Remove the needle from the arm or activate the safety shield that will remove the needle from the arm.

23. Activate the safety shield on the needle depending on the type of butterfly used.

24. Apply pressure to the site for 3 to 5 minutes. The patient may assist if able. The arm should be elevated to reduce blood flow.

25. Dispose of the needle and holder in a sharps container. When disposing, insert the needle end of the device first and allow the tubing and holder to drop into the container.

26. Recheck the identification bracelet with the labels or requisitions.

27. Label the bottles at the patient's side before leaving the examination room.

28. Label all tubes.

29. Check the puncture site. Apply adhesive bandage. If the patient is an infant, the use of the bandage should be eliminated.

30. Remove gloves and wash hands.

31. Thank the patient and transport the sample(s) to the laboratory.

Urine Collection

Procedures and standards for the collection of samples other than blood are often ignored because the patient is doing the collection. Even more time should be spent discussing these procedures with the patient so the best possible sample may be obtained. Without these instructions, the results will vary depending on how the patient collected the sample. Residue from unclean containers (anything from butter tubs to soda bottles have been used by patients) can alter results dramatically. Patient cooperation is needed for any sample to be accurate.

Urine is the most common sample to collect besides blood. The laboratory should provide the container to ensure cleanliness of the sample. For samples that are to be used for a culture, the container must be sterile (Figure 2.45). The urine can consist of a clean-catch

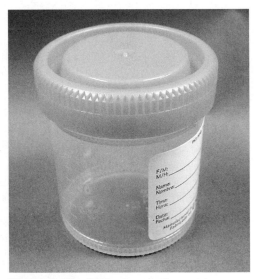

FIGURE 2.45 *Sterile urine collection container.*
© Cengage Learning 2013

midstream random sample, first morning sample, timed sample, or 24-hour sample, to name a few.

If urine testing is delayed for more than an hour after collection, special precautions must be taken. Refrigeration of the sample delays the deterioration of the sample. An alternative to refrigeration is to transfer the urine into special urine evacuated tubes that contain preservative (Figure 2.46). A urine transfer straw is inserted into the urine cup and then the evacuated tubes are filled in the same manner as a blood evacuated tube (Figure 2.47).

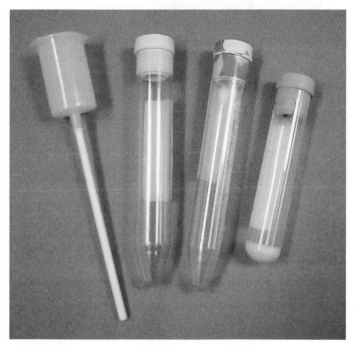

FIGURE 2.46 *Urine preservative tubes and urine transfer straw.*

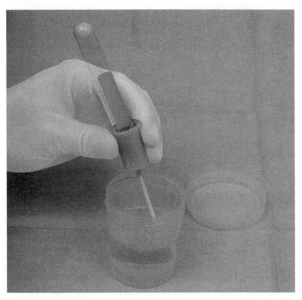

FIGURE 2.47 *The end of the straw is placed in the urine.*
© Cengage Learning 2013

The clean-catch midstream random sample is collected at any time during a 24-hour period. The patient voids in a collection container at the time the sample is needed. The patient cleans himself or herself, voids a little in the toilet, and then collects the urine sample. The procedures are slightly different depending on whether the patient is a male or female (Procedures 2.8 and 2.9). The first morning sample is collected in the same manner; it is timed to be collected when the patient first gets up in the morning.

A 24-hour collection requires the most patient cooperation. The patient voids and discards the first morning sample. All urine, including the next morning sample, is then saved in a special container supplied by the laboratory (Figure 2.48). The patient must cooperate and not

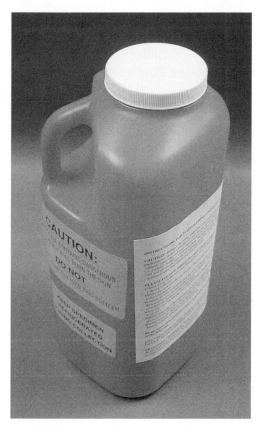

FIGURE 2.48 *Twenty-four-hour urine collection container with labels indicating that acid has been added to the container.*
© Cengage Learning 2013

discard a single sample (Procedure 2.10). Many 24-hour urine collections require that a preservative be placed into the container before collection. The patient must be notified about what the liquid in the container is and told not to pour it out.

PROCEDURE 2.8 Collecting a Clean-Catch Midstream Urine Sample: Male

Principle:

To properly and safely collect a urine sample from a male patient. The sample is a clean-catch sample taken from the midstream of the urine, collected in a sterile screw-top container.

Materials:

Gloves

Hand disinfectant

Sterile urine container

Antiseptic wipes

Label and requisition

Procedure:

1. Wash hands carefully using soap and water.
2. Using one of the antiseptic wipes, cleanse the glans (tip) of the penis. Wipe from the urethral opening (orifice), wiping from the opening in a circular motion. If you are not circumcised, this is done while holding the foreskin back. Clean the area around the opening completely. Discard the wipe.

continues

PROCEDURE 2.8 Collecting a Clean-Catch Midstream Urine Sample: Male *continued*

3. Following the first cleansing, wipe thoroughly using the second antiseptic wipe, while maintaining the foreskin in a retracted position. Discard the wipe.

4. Void a small amount of urine in the toilet bowl.

5. Continue to void and collect the urine in the cup. Do not touch the sample cup on the inside or touch your body or clothing to the cup.

6. Place the lid carefully onto the sample container. Screw the lid on tightly to prevent leakage.

7. Give the urine to the phlebotomist.

PROCEDURE 2.9 Collecting a Clean-Catch Midstream Urine Sample: Female

Principle:
To properly and safely collect a urine sample from a female patient. The sample is a clean-catch sample taken from the midstream of the urine, collected in a sterile screw-top container.

Materials:
Gloves
Hand disinfectant
Sterile urine container
Antiseptic wipes
Label and requisition

Procedure:
1. Wash hands carefully using soap and water.
2. Remove underclothing.
3. Sit comfortably on the toilet seat and swing one knee to the side as far as you can.
4. Spread the labia (outer vulva fold) with one hand and continue to keep them apart.
5. Clean the labia. Be sure to cleanse well before you collect the sample.
   a. Using an antiseptic wipe, clean one side of the fold. Using a separate towelette, clean the opposite side, wiping each time from front to back. Discard the wipes.

continues

PROCEDURE 2.9 Collecting a Clean-Catch Midstream Urine Sample: Female *continued*

    b. Using a third antiseptic wipe, wipe from the front of your body toward the back over the urethral opening. Discard the wipe.

6. Pass a small amount of urine into the toilet bowl.

7. Continue to void and collect the urine in the cup. Do not touch the sample cup on the inside or touch your body or clothing to the cup.

8. Place the lid carefully onto the sample container. Screw the lid on tightly to prevent leakage.

9. Give the urine to the phlebotomist.

PROCEDURE 2.10 Collecting a 24-hour Urine Sample

Principle:
To obtain a 24-hour urine collection, which is used to determine the 24-hour distribution of certain urine chemical output. Certain solutes exhibit diurnal variations, being higher or lower at different times of the 24-hour period. A complete 24-hour cycle shows the distribution of these variations in the total collection. Due to the length of time the urine must be collected, the urine must be refrigerated and a preservative such as hydrochloric acid may need to be added before collection.

Materials:
Gloves
Hand disinfectant
24-hour urine container
Antiseptic wipes
Additives for urine preservative
Label and requisition

Procedure:
1. Obtain a 24-hour urine sample container from the laboratory. Be careful not to touch or spill any additive that may have been placed in the container before collection.

continues

PROCEDURE 2.10 Collecting a 24-hour
Urine Sample *continued*

2. Void and discard the first morning sample and record the time.
3. Collect all urine voided during the next 24 hours. Urine should be refrigerated or kept in a cool place throughout the collection period.
4. At exactly the same time the following morning, void completely and add this sample to the container.
5. Deliver the sample to the laboratory the morning the collection was stopped. The phlebotomist will ask your name, height, weight, and the time the test was started and stopped.
6. A blood sample may also need to be collected at this time.

UNIT 3
MICROCOLLECTION

S ometimes the only alternative to collect a blood sample is to collect blood from the finger in adults or the heel in infants. Special equipment is needed to obtain accurate results when obtaining blood from the capillaries. Blood collections sometimes require capillary puncture. For this type of collection, special microcollection equipment is needed. This equipment varies in how it is used but always makes either a puncture or a cut into the skin and through the capillary bed. The equipment used to collect the blood depends on the test being performed. The equipment consists of two parts: a method of puncturing the finger or heel and a method to collect the sample.

The type of sample being collected limits the use of capillary blood collection. Certain tests require more blood than can be obtained from the capillaries.

Microcollection Equipment

Lancets

A number of different capillary puncture lancets are commercially available to puncture the skin for an adequate blood flow. Surgical blades used in the past carried the hazard of puncturing too deeply, especially in the newborn needing a heelstick or in the pediatric patient. Nonretractable lancets replaced the surgical blade and were designed for controlled depth of puncture. Nonretractable lancets consisted of a blade or needle the phlebotomist used to manually punctur the skin. The basic handheld nonretractable-blade lancets (Figure 3.1) are not used because of several disadvantages. The lancet created a hazard in that once the lancet was used on a patient, the blade was still exposed. Because the lancet was not designed to retract into a holder, as the newer style of lancets, the potential for an accidental puncture existed until the device was safely disposed of in a sharps container.

The nonretractable-blade lancet had a stop point so the phlebotomist did not stick too deep. The tendency was to be sympathetic with the patient and not stick hard enough. If this occurred, adequate blood flow was not obtained, and the patient had to be punctured again. Another disadvantage was that the patient could see the blade coming and thus became more apprehensive of the stick. Patients became so apprehensive that they would pull their hands out of the phlebotomist's grasp just as the phlebotomist was ready to stick. In a case like this, the phlebotomist would possibly stick himself or herself. The retractable

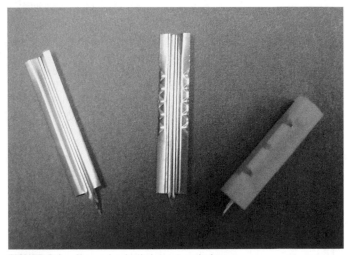

FIGURE 3.1   *Non-spring-loaded puncture devices.*
© Cengage Learning 2013

puncture device is the device now used for all capillary punctures (Figure 3.2). Multiple brands are available and are too numerous to describe in this textbook. The device will either automatically puncture the patient as it is held on his or her skin (contact-activated device) or the device is placed on the skin surface and the phlebotomist pushes the blade into the skin. With either device the blade then retracts after the puncture to prevent the phlebotomist from receiving an accidental puncture. These devices hide the blade in a plastic holder so the patient cannot see the blade during the puncture. The plastic device lies on the skin, and the blade punctures the skin. The blade then retracts. The rapid puncture and the invisible blade make the patient less apprehensive about capillary punctures. The spring-loaded blades work by a guillotine action, or a slicing motion. Devices can be purchased that puncture no more than 0.85 mm for premature infants to 2 mm for full-term newborn heelsticks. Other devices vary in depth for fingersticks of different-age patients. What should be avoided when collecting samples for laboratory tests are the devices on the market for

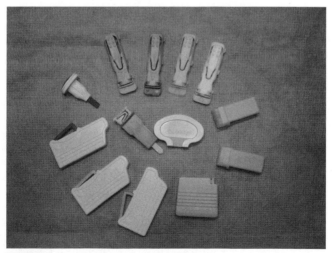

FIGURE 3.2   *Spring-loaded puncture devices.*
© Cengage Learning 2013

diabetic at-home blood glucose monitoring. These devices are excellent for their purpose but do not provide more than one or two drops of blood. This is not adequate blood flow for the sample size needed for most laboratory testing.

The devices used for collecting, processing, and transporting microcollections depend on the laboratory testing being performed. This discussion of devices here is not exhaustive. As the phlebotomist works in different laboratories, some specialized devices may also be used. Microcollection equipment is intended for one-time use to be disposed of in a sharps container.

Capillary Tubes and Microcollection Devices

The devices used for collecting, processing, and transporting microcollections depend on the laboratory testing being performed. Disposable capillary micropipettes are thin-bore devices much like small soda straws that draw the blood up to a certain line on the tubing. The line on the tubing indicates the calibration for an amount drawn from 1 to 200 microliters. They are generally used for measurement of an amount of blood and then transferred to a container or solution. The blood draws up into the tube because of capillary action. The capillary action of a tube is enhanced if the tube is slanted in a semihorizontal direction as the blood is being drawn into the tube. Plastic or plastic coating over glass is now mandated by OSHA. The glass has a tendency to break and cut the phlebotomist, exposing the phlebotomist to the patient's blood. The plastic or plastic-coated micropipettes reduce the possibility of an accidental exposure.

Microhematocrit capillary tubes are narrow-bore pipettes primarily intended for determining packed red cell volume in microsamples. Once filled, the tubes are centrifuged in a special centrifuge that packs the formed elements of the blood. This packed volume is then read on a scale that gives the packed volume as a percentage of the total. The result is the hematocrit of the patient. Because the volume is read on a special sliding scale, specific total volume in the tube is not important. The tube must be filled at least 2/3 full for accurate results. This volume required for the tube is 50 to 75 microliters.

Blood gas collection pipettes collect capillary puncture whole blood samples under anaerobic conditions for blood gas determinations. The tubes vary in size but draw 50 to 250 microliters of volume. The size of the draw needed depends on the instrument used in the blood gas testing. The tubes contain heparin to keep the blood from clotting and can be plugged with sealant putty or caps to maintain anaerobic conditions.

The process of collection and transfer of blood samples has been simplified with the use of plastic microcollection devices. These devices consist of small nonsterile plastic containers. They have included a means for filling, measuring, color-coding for the proper anticoagulant, stoppering, centrifugation, and storage. The color coding matches the coding on the anticoagulant tubes: lavender is EDTA, green is heparin, and red gives a serum sample. The serum tubes can contain the thixotropic separator gel that separates the serum or plasma from the cells after centrifugation. Bilirubin samples are collected in an amber tube that protects the blood from light. If a bilirubin sample is not protected from light, the bilirubin level of the blood in the tube will rapidly decrease.

Accurate test results require all microcollection samples be collected with a free-flowing sample. As the drop of blood forms, the collection cap, which consists of a scoop or tubing device in the cap, touches it. The blood then flows into the bottom of the tube. The tubes hold approximately 600 microliters of blood. They go by a variety of brand names, such as Microtainer and Microvette (Figure 3.3).

Capillary Puncture Blood Collection

Blood is not taken in large amounts at once from the fingerstick. It is taken in small amounts through the capillary blood flow. Blood flowing away from the heart flows in the arteries. Blood flowing back to the heart flows in the veins. Connecting most of the arteries and veins are the capillaries. Due to the one-way blood flow, the composition of the blood released from the capillary area during capillary puncture is primarily arterial blood.

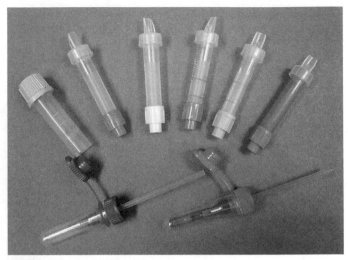

FIGURE 3.3 *Microcollection devices.*
© Cengage Learning 2013

The artery has a thick wall that helps it withstand the pressure of the pumping of the heart. The arteries branch to form arterioles that branch more to become capillaries. The capillaries then start converging to form venules, and the venules then become veins. As blood flows through the body, it follows this path of artery-capillary-vein. Oxygenated arterial blood leaves the heart and carries this oxygen to the tissue by releasing the oxygen through the cell walls of the capillaries. At the same time, carbon dioxide is being absorbed by the blood and then transported to the lungs to be exhaled as a waste product. The flow of the blood also regulates body temperature. When the body gets warm, the capillaries in the extremities dilate (enlarge in diameter) and let off heat. This process then cools the body. If the body becomes cold, the capillaries constrict (get smaller in diameter) and less blood flows through, thereby conserving heat for the rest of the body. This can be used to an advantage when collecting blood from the capillaries. Warming the site to 42°C for 3 minutes increases the blood flow by seven times. Warming can be done by using a warm washcloth, having the patient hold the hands under warm running water, or using an infant heel warmer (Figure 3.4).

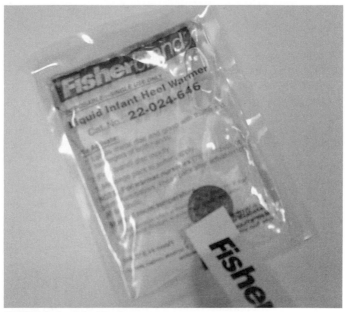

FIGURE 3.4 *Infant heel warmer.*
© Cengage Learning 2013

Obtaining a Blood Sample from a Fingerstick

Capillary puncture is the method of choice in children under 1 year old and for adults whose veins are inaccessible (Procedure 3-1). Capillary puncture is done by puncturing the skin to access the capillaries. As the patient bleeds, the blood is collected in the appropriate microcollection equipment. Adult capillary punctures are done in the finger; with children under 1 year old, the heel is the puncture site of choice.

Patients who are severely dehydrated or have poor circulation (those in shock, for example) cannot produce a capillary puncture blood sample. A patient who is extremely cold also will not produce adequate blood flow. This last situation can be rectified by warming the hand.

The site for the collection of a skin puncture in an adult is on the palmar surface of the distal phalanx of the finger. The side or tip of the finger should not be punctured because the tissue is about half as thick as the tissue in the center of the finger. The fingers of choice are the middle finger and the ring finger (second and third fingers). The puncture site must be warm or have been warmed, and the finger must not be swollen from the buildup of fluids (edematous). Puncturing an edematous finger contaminates the sample with the tissue fluid. When you puncture the finger, cut across the fingerprint line. This technique delivers the best possible blood flow and facilitates the formation of drops of blood. If the cut is made between the fingerprint lines, the fingerprints exert pressure on the cut and close the cut. The blood follows the lines of the fingerprint, resulting in no droplet formation.

Clean the finger with isopropanol (alcohol) and then dry with sterile gauze or allow to air dry thoroughly before any puncture. If the alcohol is not dry and contaminates the blood sample, the sample will become hemolyzed. Do not use povidone-iodine (Betadine) to clean and disinfect the puncture site. Even if Betadine has been allowed to thoroughly dry, it will cause elevated potassium, phosphorous, and uric acid levels.

Think before the puncture. As you hold the patient's hand, the underside of the finger may need to be the side punctured. After the puncture, the blood drips downward and gravity helps the blood flow into the collector. Before the blood sample is collected, the first drop of blood needs to be wiped away. As the finger is punctured, tissue cells are damaged, and interstitial fluid is released into the first drop. The subsequent drops are flowing due to arterial pressure.

If the puncture is adequate, 0.5 milliliter of blood can be collected from a single puncture. As the drop of blood forms at the puncture site, touch the tip of the microcollection device to the drop. Blood flow can be further enhanced by gently applying continuous pressure to the surrounding tissue. Rapid milking of the finger does not enhance the blood flow. Excess pressure may cause hemolysis or contamination of the specimen with tissue fluid.

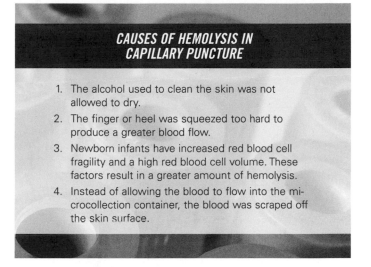

CAUSES OF HEMOLYSIS IN CAPILLARY PUNCTURE

1. The alcohol used to clean the skin was not allowed to dry.
2. The finger or heel was squeezed too hard to produce a greater blood flow.
3. Newborn infants have increased red blood cell fragility and a high red blood cell volume. These factors result in a greater amount of hemolysis.
4. Instead of allowing the blood to flow into the microcollection container, the blood was scraped off the skin surface.

Hemolysis of microcollection samples can cause inaccurate test results. Hemolysis as measured by the concentration of free hemoglobin due to ruptured red blood cells in the serum or plasma of the blood may not be readily apparent. This is particularly so in the case of those newborns with elevated bilirubin levels. The yellow of the serum may mask the red hemolysis.

Producing a sample without clots is also a challenge in microcollection. The body turns on its defenses to clot the blood at the puncture site and stop the bleeding as soon as the skin is punctured. These defenses create problems when a whole blood sample is needed. If an EDTA sample is required, the EDTA sample is drawn first to obtain an adequate volume before the blood starts to clot and platelet clumping occurs. Any other additive samples are collected next, with clotted samples last. If the blood has started to produce microscopic clots while filling the last tube, there is no problem because the blood is going to be allowed to clot in the tube.

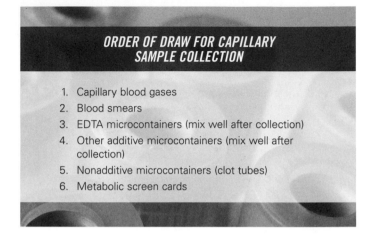

ORDER OF DRAW FOR CAPILLARY SAMPLE COLLECTION

1. Capillary blood gases
2. Blood smears
3. EDTA microcontainers (mix well after collection)
4. Other additive microcontainers (mix well after collection)
5. Nonadditive microcontainers (clot tubes)
6. Metabolic screen cards

PROCEDURE 3.1 Fingerstick Capillary Blood Collection

Principle:

To obtain capillary blood acceptable for laboratory testing as requested by a physician. The volume collected is dependent upon the test(s) ordered.

Materials:

Disposable sterile lancet

Sterile gauze squares or cotton balls

Alcohol swabs

Gloves

Sharps container

continues

PROCEDURE 3.1 Fingerstick Capillary Blood Collection
continued

Collection containers as required by test(s):

Capillary tubes

Diluting fluids

Calibrated pipettes

Microcollection containers

Glass slides

Filter paper for metabolic screen

Procedure:

1. Identify the patient. *Inpatient:* Ask the patient his or her name, to spell his or her last name, and verify the identification bracelet name and hospital number with the computer label or requisition information. *Outpatient:* Ask the patient his or her name, to spell his or her last name, and verify these with the computer label or requisition information.

2. If a fasting sample is required, ask the patient when he or she last ate. Explain the procedure to the patient.

3. Wash hands.

4. Don gloves.

5. Assemble the equipment. Select the appropriate puncture device. Select the appropriate containers for blood collection. Place the equipment within easy reach, and make any necessary preparation of fluids or containers.

6. Select the puncture site. Warm, if necessary, using a heel warmer or warm washcloth for 3 minutes.

continues

PROCEDURE 3.1 Fingerstick Capillary Blood Collection
continued

7. Finger: Use the central fleshy area of the third or fourth fingers (palmar surface of the distal phalanx of the finger).
8. Choose the finger for the puncture site that is not cold or edematous.
9. If all fingers are cold, warm the hand for 3 minutes with a warm washcloth.
10. Gently massage the finger using a milking action to increase blood flow potential (Figure 3.5).
11. Clean the puncture site with 70 percent isopropyl alcohol and let the area dry.
12. Place the puncture device firmly on the puncture site (Figure 3.6).
13. Fingerstick: The blade should be aligned to cut across the grooves of the fingerprint.
14. Puncture the skin with the disposable lancet.
15. Wipe away the first drop of blood with a sterile dry gauze or cotton ball (Figure 3.7).
16. Collect the sample in the chosen container (Figure 3.8). Touch only the tip of the collection tube to the drop of blood. Blood flow is encouraged if the puncture site is held in a downward angle and a gentle pressure applied to the finger. The order of collection is as follows:
    a. Capillary blood gases
    b. Blood smears
    c. EDTA microcontainers (mix well after collection)
    d. Other additive microcontainers (mix well after collection)

continues

PROCEDURE 3.1 Fingerstick Capillary Blood Collection
continued

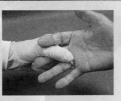

FIGURE 3.5 *Massage the finger to increase the flow of blood.*

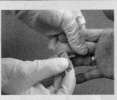

FIGURE 3.6 *Place the puncture device firmly on the puncture site.*

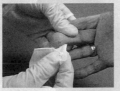

FIGURE 3.7 *Wipe away the first drop of blood.*

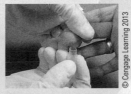

FIGURE 3.8 *Collect the sample in the chosen container.*

© Cengage Learning 2013

    e. Nonadditive microcontainers (clot tubes)

    f. Metabolic screen card

17. Seal the sample containers and immediately mix the anticoagulant tubes.

18. Apply pressure to the puncture site with a gauze square or cotton ball.

19. Label the collection containers.

20. If an insufficient sample has been obtained, the puncture may be repeated at a different site. A new sterile lancet and new collection containers must be used.

Obtaining a Blood Sample from Babies

Site Selection

Obtaining a blood microcollection sample on children under 1 year old parallels many of the same procedures as a fingerstick sample. The one main difference is the puncture site. On infants and young children, the heel is the puncture site of choice. If an infant's heel is to be punctured, the site should be on the **plantar** surface **medial** to a line drawn posteriorly from the middle of the great toe to the heel, or **lateral** to a line drawn posteriorly from between the fourth and fifth toes to the heel (Figure 3.9). In almost all infants the bones, arteries, and nerves are not near these areas. On the inside (medial, or big toe side) of the heel is the posterior tibial artery (Figure 3.10) near

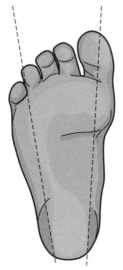

FIGURE 3.9 *Infant heel. The darkened areas illustrate the acceptable areas for puncture. The little toe side is the primary area of choice.*
© Cengage Learning 2013

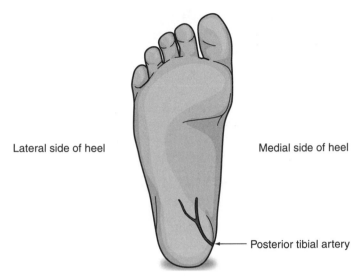

Lateral side of heel

Medial side of heel

Posterior tibial artery

FIGURE 3.10 *Infant heel, location of the posterior tibial artery.*
© Cengage Learning 2013

the curvature of the heel. The outside of the heel (lateral, or little toe side) is the area that is often suggested for use to avoid possible damage to the posterior tibial artery. This caution is unwarranted when the proper incision device is used. The controlled depth of puncture devices that are commonly used eliminates this concern. The puncture should not be done in a previous puncture site because of the possibility of infection. Do not do punctures in the central arch area of the foot. Puncture in this area may result in damage to nerves, tendons, and cartilage and offers no advantage over a heel puncture.

Depth of Puncture

The optimal depth of capillary puncture from which an adequate blood sample can be obtained without injury varies from 0.85 mm for premature infants to 2 mm for full-term infants. The capillary bed of the infant is 0.35 to 1.6 mm beneath the skin surface. A puncture of the plantar surface of the heel to a depth of 2 mm on full-term infants punctures the major capillary beds and does not injure the bone or nerves of the heel. Numerous devices are available for different ages of infants that meet the proper puncture depth depending on age.

Puncture of the fingers of infants less than 1 year old should be done only after other options are considered. The distance to the bones and main nerves of the infant's fingers is 1.2 to 2.2 mm. Many puncture devices are longer than this, and puncture of the infant's finger could result in damage to the bone or nerves with subsequent infection or permanent physical damage. The infant's finger also does not produce an adequate blood sample.

Collection of the Sample

Excessive crying of the infant can result in elevated leukocyte (white blood cell [WBC]) counts. The leukocyte count does not return to normal for up to 60 minutes. An infant who has had a procedure completed, such as circumcision, needs at least 60 minutes after crying for a blood sample to be accurate.

The procedure for microcollection from an infant is similar to that of a fingerstick on an adult or child. Procedure 3-2 details an infant heelstick procedure using a spring-loaded puncture device called a Quick Heel, manufactured by the Becton Dickinson Company.

PROCEDURE 3.2 Heelstick Capillary Puncture

Principle:
To obtain capillary blood acceptable for laboratory testing as requested by a physician.

Sample:
Capillary blood volume dependent on the test(s).

continues

PROCEDURE 3.2 Heelstick Capillary Puncture
continued

Materials:
Disposable sterile puncture device of the proper
depth for the age of the infant
Sterile gauze squares
Alcohol swabs
Gloves
Collection containers, as required by test(s):

    a. Capillary tubes

    b. Microcollection containers

    c. Calibrated pipettes

Biohazard sharps container
Safety glasses and mask

Procedure:

1. Wash hands and apply gloves before any
    patient contact.

2. Identify the patient. *Inpatient:* Check with the
    nurse to identify the patient and verify the identifi-
    cation bracelet name and hospital number with the
    computer label or requisition information. Never
    use the name on the bassinette to identify the
    infant. The information must be attached to the
    infant. Usually this is attached to the ankle of
    the infant. *Outpatient:* Ask the person bringing the
    infant in for testing to identify the infant, ask him or
    her to spell the infant's last name, and verify with
    the computer label or requisition information.

3. Verify the collection orders.

continues

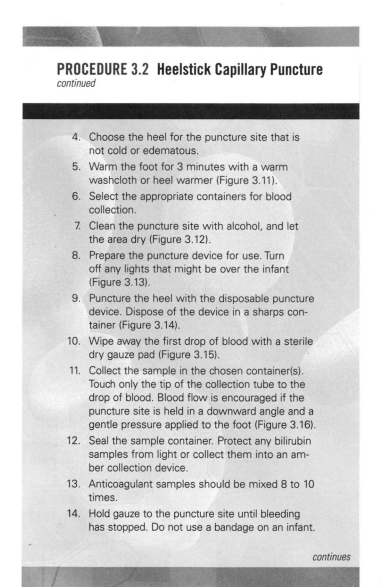

PROCEDURE 3.2 Heelstick Capillary Puncture
continued

4. Choose the heel for the puncture site that is not cold or edematous.

5. Warm the foot for 3 minutes with a warm washcloth or heel warmer (Figure 3.11).

6. Select the appropriate containers for blood collection.

7. Clean the puncture site with alcohol, and let the area dry (Figure 3.12).

8. Prepare the puncture device for use. Turn off any lights that might be over the infant (Figure 3.13).

9. Puncture the heel with the disposable puncture device. Dispose of the device in a sharps container (Figure 3.14).

10. Wipe away the first drop of blood with a sterile dry gauze pad (Figure 3.15).

11. Collect the sample in the chosen container(s). Touch only the tip of the collection tube to the drop of blood. Blood flow is encouraged if the puncture site is held in a downward angle and a gentle pressure applied to the foot (Figure 3.16).

12. Seal the sample container. Protect any bilirubin samples from light or collect them into an amber collection device.

13. Anticoagulant samples should be mixed 8 to 10 times.

14. Hold gauze to the puncture site until bleeding has stopped. Do not use a bandage on an infant.

continues

PROCEDURE 3.2 Heelstick Capillary Puncture
continued

15. Label the collection containers.
16. If an insufficient sample has been obtained, the puncture may be repeated at a different site. A new sterile lancet must be used and steps 4 to 15 must be repeated.
17. Enter the amount of the blood collected in the nursing log before returning to the laboratory.

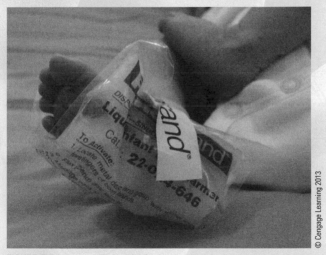

© Cengage Learning 2013

FIGURE 3.11   *Warm the heel for 3 minutes with a heel warmer.*

continues

PROCEDURE 3.2 Heelstick Capillary Puncture
continued

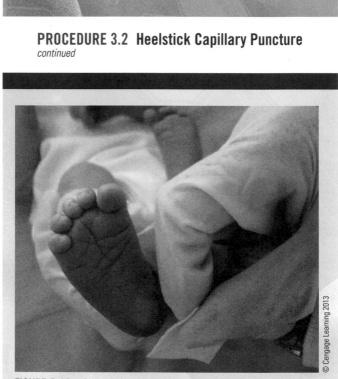

© Cengage Learning 2013

FIGURE 3.12 *Clean the incision site with an alcohol pad. Allow the alcohol to air dry. Do not touch the incision site or allow the heel to come in contact with any nonsterile item or surface.*

continues

PROCEDURE 3.2 Heelstick Capillary Puncture
continued

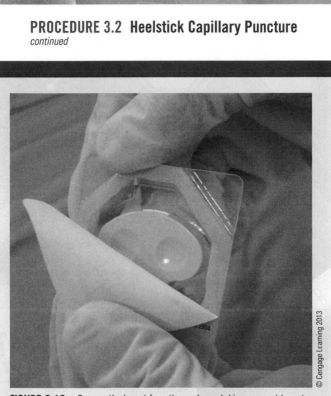

FIGURE 3.13 *Remove the lancet from the package, taking care not to rest the blade end on any nonsterile surface.*

continues

PROCEDURE 3.2 Heelstick Capillary Puncture
continued

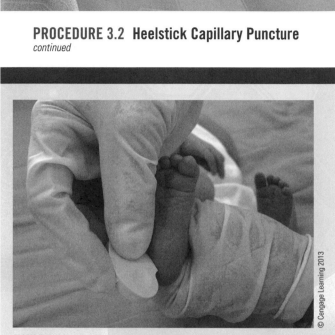

© Cengage Learning 2013

FIGURE 3.14 *Raise the foot above the baby's heart and carefully select the incision site. With gloved hand, place the blade slot area in contact with the incision area. While maintaining contact of the device with the skin, but not applying pressure, depress the plunger.*

continues

PROCEDURE 3.2 Heelstick Capillary Puncture
continued

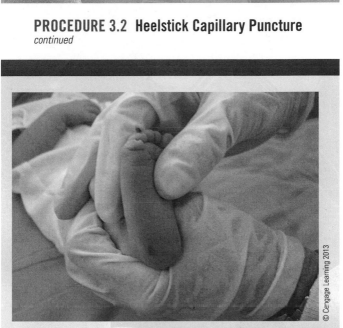

FIGURE 3.15 *After triggering, remove the lancet, discarding it in a sharps container. Using a dry gauze pad, gently wipe away the first drop of blood.*

continues

PROCEDURE 3.2 Heelstick Capillary Puncture
continued

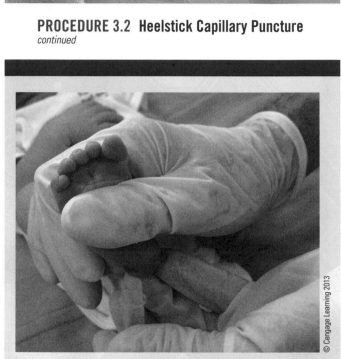

FIGURE 3.16   *Taking care not to make direct contact with the collection container, fill to the desired level. Following collection, press a clean, dry gauze pad to the incision.*

References

American Association of Blood Banks. (2008). *Technical manual* (16th ed.). Philadelphia: J. B. Lippincott.

American Diabetes Association. (2011). *Living with diabetes.* Retrieved September 2011 from http://www.diabetes.org.

Bates, D. W., Goldman, L., & Lee, T. H. (1991). Contaminant blood cultures and resource utilization: The true consequences of false-positive results. *Journal of the American Medical Association, 265,* 365–369.

Clinical Laboratory Standards Institute (CLSI). (1997). *Blood alcohol testing in the clinical laboratory; approved guideline* (CLSI Document T/DM06-A). Wayne, PA: Author.

Clinical Laboratory Standards Institute (CLSI). (2003). *Tubes and additives for venous blood specimen collection; approved standard* (5th ed.) (CLSI Document H1-A5).Wayne, PA: Author.

Clinical Laboratory Standards Institute (CLSI). (2007). *Procedures for the collection of diagnostic blood specimens by venipuncture; approved standard* (6th ed.) (CLSI Document H03-A6). Wayne, PA: Author.

Clinical Laboratory Standards Institute (CLSI). (2008). *Collection, transport, and processing of blood specimens for testing plasma-based coagulation assays and molecular hemostasis assays; approved standard* (5th ed.) (CLSI Document H21-A5). Villanova, PA: Author.

Clinical Laboratory Standards Institute (CLSI). (2008). *Procedures and devices for the collection of capillary diagnostic blood specimens; approved standard* (6th ed.) (CLSI Document H04-A6).Wayne, PA: Author.

Clinical Laboratory Standards Institute (CLSI). (2010). *Accuracy in patient and sample identification; approved guidelines* (CLSI Document GP33-A). Wayne, PA: Author.

Clinical Laboratory Standards Institute (CLSI). (2010). *Procedures for the handling and processing of blood specimens for common laboratory tests; approved standard* (4th ed.) (CLSI Document H18-A4). Wayne, PA: Author.

Guder, W. G., Narayanan, S., Wisser, H., & Zawta, B. (1996). Samples from the patient to the laboratory—the impact of preanalytical variables on the quality of laboratory results. *GIT Verlag*, Darmstadt, Germany.

Hoeltke, L. B. (1995). *The clinical laboratory manual series: Phlebotomy*. Clifton Park, NY: Delmar Cengage Learning.

Hoeltke, L. B. (2012). *The complete textbook of phlebotomy* (4th ed.). Clifton Park, NY: Delmar Cengage Learning.

Lab Tests Online. (2011). *Glucose testing*. Retrieved July 2011 from http://labtestonline.org.

Lindh, W., Pooler, M. S., Tamparo, C. D., & Cerrato, J. U. (2009). *Comprehensive medical assisting, administrative and clinical competencies*. Clifton Park, NY: Delmar Cengage Learning.

Medi-Flex Hospital Products, Inc. Cepti-Seal and ChloraPrep product literature. Overland Park, KS.

O'Hara, C. M., Weinstein, M. P., & Miller, J. M. (2007). Manual and automated systems for detection and identification of microorganisms. In P. R. Murray, E. J. Baron, J. H. Jorgensen, M. A. Pfaller, & R. H. Yoken (Eds.), *Manual of clinical microbiology* (9th ed.). Washington, DC: ASM Press.

Occupational Safety and Health Administration (OSHA). (2011). *Safety and health bulletin* (SHIB10-15-2003). Retrieved September 2011 from http://www.osha.gov.

Weinbaum, F. I., Lavie, S., Danek, M., Sixsmith, D., Heinrich, G. F., & Mills, L. S. S. (1997). Doing it right the first time: Quality improvement and the contaminant blood culture. *Journal of Clinical Microbiology, 35*(9), 563–565.

Weinstein, S., Hamrahi, V., Popat, A., Avato, I., & Gantz, N. M. (1991). Blood contamination of reusable needle holders. *American Journal of Infection Control, 19*(2).

Appendix A
Phlebotomy Competency Assessment

Phlebotomy Competency Assessment
Student/Associate: _____

Venipuncture Collection with an Evacuated Tube System

Competency: Demonstrate proper patient identification and
                sample collection technique when performing a
                venipuncture with an evacuated tube system.

Behavior: Properly identifies the patient
                Uses the appropriate collection tubes
                Follows the correct collection procedure
                Follows the order of draw

#	Task	Satisfactory Performance 2 points	Improvement Needed 1 point	Unsatisfactory Performance 0 points
1	Identifies self and the patient correctly			
2	Checks the requisition for all pertinent information			
3	Washes hands			
4	Explains the procedure to the patient			
5	Selects the correct tubes and equipment for the procedure			
6	Assembles the equipment			
7	Positions the patient's arm			
8	Ties the tourniquet			
9	Locates a vein by palpation			
10	Releases the tourniquet if needed			
11	Cleanses the site in concentric circles and allows it to air dry			

#	Task	Satisfactory Performance 2 points	Improvement Needed 1 point	Unsatisfactory Performance 0 points
12	Puts on gloves			
13	Reapplies the tourniquet if removed in step 10			
14	Positions the needle holder between the thumb and index fingers			
15	Uncaps the needle; inspects the needle for defects			
16	Anchors the vein			
17	Positions the needle at the appropriate angle			
18	Inserts the needle bevel up into the vein			
19	Collects blood following the correct order of draw			
20	Changes the tubes smoothly; does not move the needle			

#	Task	Satisfactory Performance 2 points	Improvement Needed 1 point	Unsatisfactory Performance 0 points
21	Releases the tourniquet			
22	Removes the last tube collected from the holder			
23	Covers the puncture site with gauze or a cotton ball			
24	Withdraws the needle smoothly and presses down on the gauze or cotton			
25	Activates the safety device on the needle			
26	Disposes of the needle and holder in a sharps container			
27	Inverts the tube(s) with additives several times			
28	Labels the sample(s) with the correct information			

#	Task	Satisfactory Performance 2 points	Improvement Needed 1 point	Unsatisfactory Performance 0 points
29	Checks the puncture site when the procedure is complete			
30	Disposes of used supplies in the proper containers			
31	Removes gloves and washes hands			
32	Thanks and releases the patient			
	Total points in each category			
	Total in all categories			

Student/associate signature: ＿＿＿＿＿＿＿＿   **Date:** ＿＿＿＿＿＿＿

Instructor signature: ＿＿＿＿＿＿＿＿＿＿   **Date:** ＿＿＿＿＿＿＿

Supervisor signature: ＿＿＿＿＿＿＿＿＿＿   **Date:** ＿＿＿＿＿＿＿

Phlebotomy Competency Assessment
Student/Associate: _____

Venipuncture Collection with a Butterfly Needle

Competency: Demonstrate proper patient identification and sample collection technique when performing a venipuncture with a butterfly needle.

Behavior: Properly identifies the patient
Uses the appropriate collection tubes
Follows the correct collection procedure
Follows the order of draw

#	Task	Satisfactory Performance 2 points	Improvement Needed 1 point	Unsatisfactory Performance 0 points
1	Identifies self and the patient correctly			
2	Checks the requisition for all pertinent information			
3	Washes hands			
4	Explains the procedure to the patient			
5	Selects the correct tubes and equipment for the procedure			

#	Task	Satisfactory Performance 2 points	Improvement Needed 1 point	Unsatisfactory Performance 0 points
6	Assembles the equipment			
7	Positions the patient's arm			
8	Ties the tourniquet			
9	Locates a vein by palpation			
10	Releases the tourniquet if needed			
11	Cleanses the site in concentric circles and allows it to air dry			
12	Puts on gloves			
13	Reapplies the tourniquet if removed in step 10			
14	Holds the butterfly by the wings			
15	Uncaps the needle; inspects the needle for defects			
16	Anchors the vein			

#	Task	Satisfactory Performance 2 points	Improvement Needed 1 point	Unsatisfactory Performance 0 points
17	Positions the needle at the appropriate angle			
18	Inserts the needle bevel up into the vein			
19	Collects blood following the correct order of draw			
20	Changes the tubes smoothly; does not move the needle			
21	Releases the tourniquet			
22	Removes the last tube collected from the holder			
23	Covers the puncture site with gauze or a cotton ball			
24	Withdraws the needle smoothly and presses down on the gauze or cotton			

#	Task	Satisfactory Performance 2 points	Improvement Needed 1 point	Unsatisfactory Performance 0 points
25	Activates the safety device on the butterfly			
26	Disposes of the needle and holder in a sharps container			
27	Inverts the tube(s) with additives several times			
28	Labels the sample(s) with the correct information			
29	Checks the puncture site when the procedure is complete			
30	Disposes of used supplies in the proper containers			
31	Removes gloves and washes hands			
32	Thanks and releases the patient			

#	Task	Satisfactory Performance 2 points	Improvement Needed 1 point	Unsatisfactory Performance 0 points
	Total points in each category			
	Total in all categories			

Student/associate signature: _____ **Date:** _____

Instructor signature: _____ **Date:** _____

Supervisor signature: _____ **Date:** _____

Phlebotomy Competency Assessment
Student/Associate: _____

Blood Culture Butterfly Collection

Competency: Demonstrate proper patient identification and
sample collection technique when collecting a
blood culture.

Behavior: Properly identifies the patient
Uses the appropriate blood culture collection
bottles
Follows the correct collection procedure
Follows the order of draw

#	Task	Satisfactory Performance 2 points	Improvement Needed 1 point	Unsatisfactory Performance 0 points
1	Identifies self and the patient correctly			
2	Checks the requisition for all pertinent information			
3	Washes hands			
4	Explains the procedure to the patient			
5	Selects the correct tubes, blood culture bottles, and equipment for the procedure			

#	Task	Satisfactory Performance 2 points	Improvement Needed 1 point	Unsatisfactory Performance 0 points
6	Assembles the butterfly needle and special blood culture holder			
7	Cleanses the tops of blood culture bottles with alcohol			
8	Positions the patient's arm			
9	Ties the tourniquet			
10	Locates a vein by palpation			
11	Releases the tourniquet if needed			
12	Cleanses the site in concentric circles with the blood culture prep kit and allows it to air dry			
13	Puts on gloves			
14	Reapplies the tourniquet if removed in step 10			

#	Task	Satisfactory Performance 2 points	Improvement Needed 1 point	Unsatisfactory Performance 0 points
15	Holds the butterfly by the wings			
16	Uncaps the needle; inspects the needle for defects			
17	Anchors the vein			
18	Positions the needle at the appropriate angle			
19	Inserts the needle bevel up into the vein			
20	Collects blood following the correct order of draw; aerobic blood culture bottle is collected first			
21	Changes the bottles/tubes smoothly; does not move the needle			
22	Releases the tourniquet			

#	Task	Satisfactory Performance 2 points	Improvement Needed 1 point	Unsatisfactory Performance 0 points
23	Removes the last tube collected from the holder			
24	Covers the puncture site with gauze or a cotton ball			
25	Withdraws the needle smoothly and presses down on the gauze or cotton			
26	Activates the safety device on the butterfly			
27	Disposes of the needle and holder in a sharps container			
28	Inverts the tube(s) with additives several times			
29	Labels the sample(s) with the correct information			

#	Task	Satisfactory Performance 2 points	Improvement Needed 1 point	Unsatisfactory Performance 0 points
30	Checks the puncture site when the procedure is complete			
31	Disposes of used supplies in the proper containers			
32	Removes gloves and washes hands			
33	Thanks and releases the patient			
	Total points in each category			
	Total in all categories			

Student/associate signature: _____ Date: _____

Instructor signature: _____ Date: _____

Supervisor signature: _____ Date: _____

Phlebotomy Competency Assessment
Student/Associate: _____

Capillary Skin Puncture Collection

Competency: Demonstrate proper patient identification and
sample collection technique when performing a
capillary blood collection.

Behavior: Properly identifies the patient
Uses the appropriate lancet device and collection
tubes
Follows the correct collection procedure
Follows the order of draw

#	Task	Satisfactory Performance 2 points	Improvement Needed 1 point	Unsatisfactory Performance 0 points
1	Identifies self and the patient correctly			
2	Checks the requisition for all pertinent information			
3	Washes hands			
4	Explains the procedure to the patient			
5	Selects the correct lancet, tubes, and equipment for the procedure			

#	Task	Satisfactory Performance 2 points	Improvement Needed 1 point	Unsatisfactory Performance 0 points
6	Assembles the equipment			
7	Puts on gloves			
8	Selects the site for capillary puncture			
9	Applies the warmer to the site if appropriate			
10	Cleanses the site and allows it to air dry			
11	Secures the puncture site to avoid patient movement			
12	Performs the puncture smoothly			
13	Disposes of the lancet in the sharps container			
14	Wipes away the first drop of blood			
15	Collects rounded drops into collection container without scraping the blood			

#	Task	Satisfactory Performance 2 points	Improvement Needed 1 point	Unsatisfactory Performance 0 points
16	Does not squeeze too vigorously			
17	Collects an adequate amount of blood			
18	Follows the correct order of draw			
19	Mixes the collection containers when appropriate			
20	Cleanses the site and applies pressure			
21	Labels the sample(s) with the correct information			
22	Checks the puncture site on the patient			
23	Covers the puncture site with bandage if applicable			
24	Removes gloves and washes hands			

#	Task	Satisfactory Performance 2 points	Improvement Needed 1 point	Unsatisfactory Performance 0 points
25	Thanks and releases the patient			
	Total points in each category			
	Total in all categories			

Student/associate signature: _____ Date: _____

Instructor signature: _____ Date: _____

Supervisor signature: _____ Date: _____

Appendix B
Phlebotomy Test Questions

Multiple-Choice Questions

1. The gauge of the needle indicates the following relationship—the larger the gauge number, the
   a. larger the diameter of the bore.
   b. longer the needle.
   c. shorter the needle.
   d. smaller the diameter of the bore.

2. If the blood is drawn too quickly from a vein, the vein will have a tendency to
   a. bruise.
   b. collapse.
   c. disintegrate.
   d. roll.

3. The bevel of the needle
   a. attaches to the syringe or the holder.
   b. should be held at a 50-degree angle to the skin.
   c. should always be facing up when inserted into the skin.
   d. should always be facing down when inserted into the skin.

4. In which of the following conditions would you avoid a site for venipuncture?
   a. edematous arm
   b. arm with IV
   c. hematoma
   d. all of the above

5. In drawing blood samples, which of the following should be performed first?
   a. Clean the site.
   b. Find the vein.
   c. Apply the tourniquet.
   d. Identify the patient.

6. What is the major drawback of a 24-hour urine collection?
   a. The tests done are unreliable.
   b. Preservatives must be used.
   c. Doctors do not know when to order it.
   d. Patient cooperation is essential and often hard to get.

7. The components of blood found inside of a tube drawn with anticoagulant are
   a. plasma, buffy coat, and erythrocytes.
   b. buffy coat and clot.
   c. serum and buffy coat.
   d. serum and clot.

8. Venipuncture is usually performed in the anticubital area. Which vein is *usually* the best to draw from?
   a. cephalic
   b. basilic
   c. median cubital
   d. none of the above

9. The gray-stoppered tube is usually drawn for which test?
   a. glucose
   b. PTT

c. enzyme

d. hematology

10. The doctor orders a CBC (lavender stopper), comprehensive metabolic panel (SST), PT (light-blue stopper), and a set of blood cultures. What is the order of draw?

    a. SST tube, light blue, blood culture, lavender

    b. blood culture, light blue, lavender, SST

    c. blood culture, light blue, SST, lavender

    d. blood culture, green, light blue, SST

11. What can happen if the tourniquet is left on too long before drawing blood?

    a. hematoma

    b. hemolysis

    c. hemoconcentration

    d. none of the above

12. The formed elements make up about ___ of the whole blood volume.

    a. 30 percent

    b. 45 percent

    c. 55 percent

    d. 60 percent

13. Which of the following statements is NOT true?

    a. Gray-stoppered tubes are used for blood glucose tests.

    b. Gray-stoppered tubes are used for CBC and WBC tests.

    c. Lavender-stoppered tubes are used for CBC, WBC, and platelet testing.

    d. Red-stoppered tubes are used for many tests, including serum enzyme testing.

14. The depth of cut made by a lancet for a heelstick on a full-term infant should be NO MORE THAN

    a. 1.5 millimeters.

    b. 2 millimeters.

    c. 2.8 millimeters.

    d. 3 millimeters.

15. The single most important way to prevent the spread of infection in a hospital or other health care facility is

    a. gowning and gloving.

    b. handwashing.

    c. always wearing gloves.

    d. avoiding breathing on patients.

16. The tourniquet should not be left on more than ___ minute(s) before a flow of blood is obtained.

    a. 1

    b. 4

    c. 6

    d. 10

17. As a general rule, you should not stick a person more than ___ in an attempt to obtain blood.

    a. once

    b. twice

    c. three times

    d. four times

18. What is the best sample for urine collection?

    a. any random sample

    b. a catheterized sample

    c. a clean-catch midstream urine sample

    d. a sample from an ostomy bag

19. The most common cause of blood culture contamination is

    a. collection of too much blood.

    b. collection of the sample from below the IV.

    c. improper skin preparation.

    d. use of a needle and syringe for collection.

20. Serum is described as hemolyzed in the presence of increased
    a. bilirubin, causing jaundice
    b. carbon dioxide from cell metabolism
    c. hemoglobin due to ruptured RBCs
    d. lipids in a nonfasting sample

21. Why must the first drop of blood from a capillary puncture be wiped away?
    a. to remove interstitial (tissue) fluid
    b. to wipe away any bacterial contamination
    c. to remove heparin/saline contamination
    d. to make the blood flow faster

22. Which of the following items are minimum requirements for sample labeling?
    a. patient's complete name, identification number, date, time of collection, and physician
    b. patient's complete name, identification number, date, time of collection, and collector's initials
    c. patient's complete name and identification number
    d. patient's complete name, date, and time of collection

23. When serum is needed for testing, blood should be collected in which color stoppered tube?
    a. light blue
    b. green
    c. lavender
    d. red

24. The anticoagulant preferred for hematology testing is
    a. citrate.
    b. EDTA.
    c. fluoride.
    d. heparin.

Matching Questions

    a. glass red-stoppered tube
    b. light blue–stoppered tube
    c. green-stoppered tube
    d. lavender-stoppered tube
    e. gray-stoppered tube
    f. plastic SST tube

25. _____ Contains no additive
26. _____ Contains glycolytic inhibitor (prevents glycolysis)
27. _____ Preserves the cell morphology for a differential
28. _____ Contains EDTA
29. _____ Requires a 1:9 ratio
30. _____ Contains a clot activator
31. _____ Contains heparin
32. _____ Contains oxalate
33. _____ Contains thixotropic gel
34. _____ Gives a serum sample (two answers)
35. _____ Gives a serum sample (two answers)

Critical Thinking Questions

1. Explain the difference between serum and plasma tubes. Find tubes in the laboratory that represent each type of tube.
2. A patient indicates he has a latex allergy. Explain the changes in equipment you would need to make to accommodate this patient.
3. You draw two light blue–stoppered tubes on a patient and both tubes fill only half full. What would be the problem if you poured the two tubes together to make a full tube, as you know is required with a light blue–stoppered tube?
4. Explain the difference between a glass red-stoppered tube and a plastic red-stoppered tube in the ability of the tube to clot.

5. The patient has an IV running in her right hand. The left arm is in a cast, so you go to the only available site, in the median cubital vein of the right arm, to collect your blood sample. The IV is running a saline solution, and you are going to collect a sample for glucose testing. You assume there will not be a problem. Are you correct?

Answers to Questions

1. d
2. b
3. c
4. d
5. d
6. d
7. a
8. c
9. a
10. c
11. c
12. b
13. b
14. b
15. b
16. a
17. b
18. c
19. c
20. c
21. a
22. b
23. d
24. b

25. a
26. e
27. d
28. d
29. b
30. f
31. c
32. e
33. f
34. a
35. f

Answers to Critical Thinking Questions

1. Serum tubes are tubes that are going to allow the blood within the tube to clot; therefore, after centrifugation the liquid portion will be serum. A plasma tube has an anticoagulant chemical in the tube to prevent the blood from clotting. The liquid portion from this tube is plasma.

    Some examples of serum tubes are: red stoppered, gold stoppered, red/black stoppered. Examples of plasma tubes are: light-blue stoppered, lavender stoppered, gray stoppered, green stoppered.

2. If a patient indicates having a latex allergy you will need to clean the area that the patient will have contact with, such as the chair and arm of the drawing chair. Wash your hands and use a latex-free tourniquet, latex-free gloves, and latex-free bandages.

3. The light blue–stoppered tube must be full with the proper blood-to-anticoagulant ratio. By pouring the two half-filled tubes together you are doubling the anticoagulant and offsetting the proper ratio.

4. Both a glass and plastic red-stoppered tube will clot the blood. The plastic red-stoppered tube needs the have a clot activator within the tube in order for the blood to clot.

5. Collecting blood from the arm that has a saline IV running will dilute the blood sample with saline solution. This will give an inaccurate result for the glucose test.

Index